Yoga and Diet Cured My Arthritis

Includes a 14-day diet and exercise plan towards recovery
and Mysore Ashtanga Yoga Practice Manual

Mark Flint
2017
KPJAYI Authorised Teacher

Dedicated to the Angels I have met on my journey.

D1550720

FOREWORD

Arthritis is a condition that many people live with – with varying degrees of pain and decreased mobility in the effected limbs. The term covers any disorder that affects the joints. It is a multifaceted condition that expresses itself in numerous ways and the cause or causes are still not well understood. So far, medical science has not come up with a total cure.

More than 20 years ago I decided to seek my own methods of relieving the symptoms of my rheumatoid arthritis – one of the more debilitating forms of the dis-ease - rather than succumb to a lifetime regime of medication and restrictions, which come with their own sets of consequences.

The first part of this book describes that journey and the new way of living that I learnt along the way. I have changed almost everything in my life but the result has been good health and wellbeing. I then discuss what I have found out about the various kinds of arthritis and the commonly used ways medicos treat the symptoms.

In the following sections of the book I share with you the alternative methods I have found through my own experience that alleviated my symptoms and restored my general health to the extent that I now feel 'cured'. However, I have also found that if I stray too far from the practices that work for me, the dis-ease is likely to flare up again.

I learnt that the foods you eat can have a strong effect. So I developed an approach to diet that will help you to eliminate those foods that have a negative affect and increase those which have a positive result for you. I then provide lists of healthy food sources so you can design your own menus.

Throughout my journey I tried many exercise regimes to maintain and increase joint mobility and control pain or discomfort with varying degrees of success. Discovering Yoga over 20 years ago was a turning point for me. Consistent practice of the asanas has increased my mobility. Even if you can only complete the movements in 'Basic Ashtanga Yoga for Arthritic Relief' in Section 5 you will benefit.

On going recovery from arthritis depends on forming new habits. The new habits may be daily medication and avoiding certain movements or activities or they may be habits that change your way of life and introduce new ways of managing your body. When I reflect on my life now I almost feel grateful for the dis-ease that has led me to a more fulfilling and happy lifestyle than I ever imagined. I hope the same for you.

Mark Flint 1st January 2017.

Yoga and Diet Cured My Arthritis

Yoga and Diet Cured My Arthritis
Includes a 14-day diet and exercise plan towards recovery
and Mysore Ashtanga Yoga Practice Manual

First published in 2017 by Yorkshire Buddha
Text copyright Mark Flint 2017-01-29
Photography and edit credits to:
Cover photo Immo Nykanen
Back cover Alessandro Sigismondi
Asana photos.chinayogaonline.com
Modified photos Andre B C Drottholm
Photo Editing Charlot Kryza
Text Edit Suzy McKenna

Published by Yorkshire Buddha

DISCLAIMER

The views, opinions and advice given in this book are based on the personal experiences of the author, who is not a qualified mainstream health practitioner.

The author disclaims any liabilities or loss in connection with the exercises, diet and any other information or advice herein. If you have a persistent health problem you should consult a health practitioner.

Please be aware that not all yoga exercises are suitable for everyone straight away and it takes time to be able to complete all the asanas. When you have completed suryanamaskar A & B the author suggests you find a competent and qualified teacher to help you further with the primary series of asanas.

Table of Contents

SECTION 1: MY STORY

I am 54 years young at the time of writing this book. Currently, I live in Mysore, India with my wife Stephanie and beautiful child Oliver. We are committed students of ashtanga yoga at the Krishna Pattabhi Jois Ashtanga Yoga Institute (KPJAYI). Stephanie and I are both KP-JAYI authorized teachers and we travel 3 to 4 months every year teaching yoga workshops in Asia and Europe.

In Mysore we run 'Shanti Nilayam', a heritage guesthouse catering to some of the thousands of yogis who come to Mysore on their yoga pilgrimage. We also own 'Mysore Yoga Accessories' producing yoga and therapeutic aids that we export globally.

As a ten-year-old child I was a dedicated, serious golfer and turned professional at the young age of 16. At age 18 I decided to give up my golfing career for personal not health reasons. Golf gave me so much but I felt much more was out there in the bigger world.

Then when I was 30 years old I started experiencing pain and swelling in my fingers and toe joints. I went to the local doctor who referred me to a rheumatoid arthritis specialist at a city hospital. The physician was highly regarded in his field and was ranked among the top three specialists in the country. I went to the appointment even though I had already met this doctor socially and knew at this point I did not did not hold him in high regard.

After a few visits and several tests I was finally diagnosed with rheumatoid arthritis and told I should start a long-term (lifetime) course of medication including steroids, painkillers and anti-inflammatories. I questioned the doctor about this, mentioning I had read about research by a team of Scandinavian scientists finding that rheumatoid arthritis was directly linked to diet. He replied that there was no evidence to prove that theory and if I did not take his advice and his steroids I would slowly deteriorate and eventually become crippled and spend my life in a wheelchair. I bid him farewell, refusing his prescription, and left his office for the last time.

His words scared me. I was 30 years old, an ex-professional sportsman with a passion for life. To the outside world I looked fit, strong and athletic but inside the pain at times was excruciating. I went on my own course of self-discovery and even stopped taking Ibuprofen unless absolutely necessary. I saw the pain as my body's warning signal that something needed to be addressed.

I already had a little knowledge of karma and Eastern philosophy. From an early age, I often doodled the symbols for Aum and Yin Yang without knowing where these images came from or why they were so prominent and always with me.

A friend told me about how he had suffered from arthritis in the knee and was successfully treated with acupuncture. I immediately found an acupuncturist in a nearby town and arranged a consultation. This particular doctor was British but had grown up in India. His consultation room was like a wizard's den complete with a skeleton, prosthetics and pictures of body maps. Upon speaking with him I soon realized I had found a different style of medical professional who was prepared to listen to me, answer any questions I had, explain my disease and share his knowledge. I signed up for a course of treatments but unfortunately acupuncture did not work for me. However, I gained some valuable knowledge about pain gateways and diet. I also learnt from him that allopathic medicines simply suppressed the symptoms of the disease, whereas alternative therapies worked at curing the disease by eradicating it from the body through identification and removal of the underlying cause.

In 2006 I undertook a diploma in Clinical Acupuncture with the late Anton Jayasuria in Sri Lanka where I successfully treated arthritic patients in the clinic with acupuncture, along with oil manipulation and apple cider vinegar tonic. One elderly lady who had suffered from pain and inflammation in her knees was overjoyed when the treatment worked and she could walk freely again. I was touched by this and knew I was doing something right.

I realized, through these experiences, that what works for some people might not be right for others; this includes alternative therapies and food.

I learned that by keeping a diary of what you consume and its effects, you can find out what is beneficial or harmful to you as an individual.

I continued research into diet and started recording what was good for me and what was bad. I also heard about gout, the so-called rich man's disease that is brought about by consuming rich foods, red meats, shellfish, wine, port and brandy etc. I was living quite a decadent life at the time and noticed that some of these foods were having a noticeable effect on my condition and exaggerating the symptoms. I also discovered that some vegetables in the solanaceae or nightshade family (such as potatoes and capsicums), along with processed and fast foods were influencing the conditions of my disease.

We are told "you are what you eat" but we do not adhere to this dictum in the face of modern food choices. We can actually eat to cure dis-ease (this also works on cancers and other diseases). You can eat yourself back to good health by eating the correct foods that naturally combat a disease. Eating foods that are fresh and contain the correct balance of nutrients will help keep your body healthy while eating processed food can have the opposite effect.

It was around this time the world was waking up to the harmful effects of additives and preservatives in packaged food (identified by E numbers on the packaging). A few were eventually banned but many remained.

I noticed processed foods were having a very negative effect on my body so I decided to restrict consumption of them and the toxins they contain. I remembered that when I was a boy a brand of processed orange juice made me run around like an overactive child. Today I would have been diagnosed with attention deficit and hyperactivity disorder (ADHD) and put on a course of medication to suppress it, not acknowledging that it was caused by something that I had consumed. Some doctors are now more accepting of diet as a major contributing factor in ADHD and other diseases but they still keep prescribing harmful drugs instead of recommending a corrective controlled diet that avoids processed and fast foods.

Winters and the cold weather were the worst times for me. Like many others, I found it difficult to walk in the mornings and had severe pain if I accidentally knocked my hands. I had been paying high health insurance premiums for many years and eventually I made a claim for a disability allowance, as I was not able to continue my work. The claim was investigated and rejected because I could still answer the phone, which was considered an integral part of my job, and because I had refused the physician's recommended medicine! To the outside world I still appeared normal, but inside the pain was constant. I felt the whole system was against me: the insurance company, the drug companies, and the national health system. But I was not prepared to give in.

Back in the mid-80s I had a friend who was one of the early teachers of the Alexander Technique. She introduced me to her art and I was amazed about the harm we were doing to our bodies through the bad posture that we have slowly adopted in our search to make life easier.

Simply by the way we use chairs we are doing everything wrong: we don't use the spine, legs or head correctly, weight is unevenly disbursed, and our centre of gravity is altered. I now try to be conscious of those early discoveries and put them into practice. I often compare Alexander Technique with the teaching of B.K.S. Iyengar, both the teachings of very gifted individuals who went on their own course of self-discovery, observing and understanding the human body and becoming masters of their own body and health.

I had developed a passing interest in yoga, but there were very few classes to be found in the United Kingdom at that time. Yoga was either a hippie thing practiced by remnants of the 1960s who had done the overland experience to India, or coffee morning yoga for the over 50s.

I never found a suitable class but I did have an Indian friend who taught me some simple stretches and sitting postures that he had learned from his grandfather when he was a child. It was very different from the ashtanga yoga I practice and teach now. My friend could easily sit in padmasana (lotus position), something in the West we see as a great challenge. I started learning these simple stretches. It felt good but I knew there had to be more.

In 1998 I took my second trip to India. The first trip had been a beach holiday in Goa. This time I travelled for over a month in this incredible, diverse country. I landed in Delhi in winter, it was cold and very polluted but there was a special type of magic in the air. I travelled a little in the north then worked my way down to the south. Bangalore was a fast and growing city, eagerly meeting the demands of the booming IT sector. I visited Coorge in the Western Ghats, famous for producing most of India's coffee, with its mountains, lush jungles and rainforest. Then I went on to Mysore and planned to go to Hampi to end the vacation. When I landed in Mysore I instantly felt something very special.

The city carries many tags: 'Retirement paradise of India'; 'Garden City;' 'City of Palaces'. It is the old state capital of Karnataka and the seat of the Wadiyar Empire. The Mysore Maharaja Krishnaraja Wadiyar III had been reinstated as ruler of the state when the British defeated the Muslim warlord Tipu Sultan and his French battalion in a bloody battle at Srirangapatna on the outskirts of the city. The Wadiyars were deeply loved by their subjects, building the first hydro-electric dam in Asia and providing irrigation canals for agriculturists. They also built many educational institutions that still bear the family name. Krishnarajendra Wadiyar IV was a patron of the arts and very much a 'Europhile' welcoming many European travellers and dignitaries to Mysore. The city is well planned with beautiful public buildings built in Georgian style and a magnificent palace in the centre of the city.

Mysore has a temperate climate with highs of 38 degrees and lows of 18 degrees throughout the year with little humidity. It has a very light monsoon and is surrounded by beautiful nature, crafted paddy fields, mountains, rainforest and jungle. I did not know when I arrived that it was also the home of ashtanga yoga as taught by Sri K Pattabhi Jois following the lineage of T. Krishnamacharya, the father of modern yoga. T. Krishnamacharya taught in Mysore at Jaganmohan palace under the patronage of the Maharaja Krishnarajendra Wadiyar IV through the 1930s and 40s.

More important for me at that time was that Mysore had a good golf course, great weather, nature and beautiful architecture. I extended my stay for 2 more days and didn't go to Hampi. Instead I investigated the city further, met some real estate agents and got a general idea of the price of property and living standards.

I returned to England and decided I was going to sell everything and move to Mysore. Eight months later my tickets were booked to depart in October 1999. With my possessions packed into a shipping container, 'the India adventure was starting'.

My friends thought I was crazy. Their impression of India was of a poor, destitute, third world country. Bangalore, the neighbouring city to Mysore and the present state capital of Karnataka, was still pretty much unknown outside of IT circles, but is now known all over the world as the Silicon Valley of India.

I arrived in Mysore and was living in a hotel while searching for a house. On the second day I started a yoga course at the city's Ayurvedic Hospital on Sayaji Rao Rd. This turned out not to be the style of yoga for me but I learned from it what I could and continued my search. After experimenting with different teachers and styles I eventually found my first 'Yoga Guru': he was a young and very gifted practitioner by the name of Shiva Kumar, a star student of Acharya Venkatesh and for 9 years national yoga asana champion of India.

I was his first international student and I was grateful to be given his personal attention. Under his tutorship I started to learn the intricacies of hatha yoga. One sad day he informed me he had been offered a teaching appointment abroad and would be leaving India, I had lost my teacher. I continued with self-practice and tried some more Indian teachers but I could not find anyone to take the place of my young Guru.

By this time I was familiar with Sri K. Pattabhi Jois and ashtanga yoga but I was ill informed about the practice. I heard that it was too strong and people easily got injured. I now know the truth: that it is not the ashtanga system that breaks you; it is your own ego.

I started practicing the ashtanga series, which I had learned from friends, but I was not doing vinyasa and I skipped the asanas I thought I could not do.

In another milestone in my life, my UK business partner went bankrupt and then my main Indian product supplier refused to pay me my earned commissions. It was 2008 and the world was experiencing another economic slowdown so I decided to take a six- month sabbatical from business and dedicate more time to yoga. I had met both Sharath and his grandfather Pattabhi Jois on several occasions and decided to visit Sharath at KPJAYI and ask if I could be his student. He accepted me, his only condition was that I would be committed to a regular daily practice - I agreed.

I joined the afternoon class for Indian students under his personal supervision and soon realized I had again found my yoga guru. In a short time he had me doing the complete primary series including the asanas I had shied away from and thought I could not do.

The six months I had allocated passed quickly and I became addicted to ashtanga yoga, I had found my practice and I never looked back; yoga became a way of life. I was granted the blessing to teach in 2012 by KPJAYI and joined a select few authorized teachers worldwide of this traditional ashtanga yoga system.

I now travel three to four months each year teaching workshops and spend the remaining months in Mysore practicing under the guidance of my teacher.

In addition to exploring the effects of diet and regular yoga practice on arthritis symptoms, my journey also involved exploring meditation and alternative health therapies.

After the loss of my father in 2001 I had joined an organization that practices meditation as a route to salvation. Soon I was meditating 5 hours per day. While this sounds excessive, previously I would sleep for 10 hours. After starting to meditate I brought sleep time down to 5 hours and meditation up to 5 hours. My life was transformed. I felt pure and cleansed like never before.

Even though I left that organization I did learn some very valuable lessons that I still use to this day, I still meditate when I feel the need and have participated in Vipassana and Zen meditation programs.

I have not been totally clean with my lifestyle choices, sometimes playing Russian roulette with the disease, knowing that sometimes I may get an adverse reaction to certain things. But through this I have also found my tolerance levels and noticed they have changed to certain things over the years. What gave me an adverse reaction before does not necessarily induce an adverse reaction now. One thing I have maintained is to avoid all processed foods.

In over 20 years I have had only a handful of severe attacks. These were mostly self- inflicted or related to a major stress event in my life. A couple of times I have given into mainstream medications for a quick fix but for no longer than a few days.

During one attack I was using Ibuprofen to take down the swelling and mask the pain but I had an allergic reaction to it causing my liver to swell.

I had met a local homeopathic, nature cure doctor, familiarly called Dr Jag, who practices his own mix of natural treatments with huge success. He spends half the year at his free clinic in Mysore and the other half in Brunei. He treated me with oil manipulation and told me to continue this regime morning, noon and evening. He also suggested I should take apple cider vinegar with honey and a little water in the morning and evening and I should drink a celery leaf or dandelion leaf infusion instead of tea or coffee to improve my circulation. Within a few days under his care I was back to normal.

Dr Jag is famous for lecturing people about their eating habits and recommends drastic diet changes that sometimes are hard for people to follow, but this is the route to cure and he leaves them with that choice. I will always thank him for helping me and confirming I was on the right path to tackle my dis-ease.

When I first heard the term 'disease modifying anti-rheumatic drugs' I was curious, so I booked an appointment to see the top rheumatoid arthritis specialist in Bangalore. I was honest with him and told him my disease history and my choice to refuse allopathic medicine and take a different approach to the disease. One of the first things he said to me was that by seeing the deformity in the hands he could guess I was suffering from gout and not rheumatoid arthritis. After taking blood tests it was confirmed I was both gout and rheumatoid arthritis positive. The doctors in the UK had not diagnosed this or it could be something that developed later. For me it answered a lot of questions about diet and its contributing factors to the dis-ease.

The doctor explained the latest advances in the use of 'disease modifying anti-rheumatic drugs' but he did not try to convince me to use them. He also confirmed that I was managing to control the disease and should continue my own choice of treatment.

SECTION 2: ARTHRITIS

Arthritis means 'inflammation of the joints'. 'Arthro' refers to joints and 'itis' refers to inflammation. Arthritis is not discriminatory; it can affect people of all ages. It is not one single disease and has many different factors, the most common being pain and inflammation of the joints.

The different types of arthritis include: rheumatoid arthritis, osteoarthritis, gout, Still's disease, spondylitis, traumatic arthritis and neurogenic joint disease.

The Arthritis Foundation runs a website with up-to-date and in depth information about the various kinds of arthritis and both medical and everyday or alternative ways of dealing with it. It is a great resource for people with arthritis and gout.

http://www.arthritis.org/about-arthritis/

Experts are not settled on the cause or causes of arthritis, but I believe from years of study and experimentation with my own symptoms that the key underlying factors are excess uric acid in the body and an immune system that is not working correctly. Other contributing factors include an imbalance of toxins due to bad diet and wrong food combinations. In addition, hormone imbalance, emotional stress and repetitive stress syndrome may also be contributing factors.

Some foods produce a lot of uric acid, while over-cooking food destroys the alkaline salts that are essential to neutralise acid in the body. When too much uric acid is present in the body it gets carried round the system by the blood and it is deposited in the joints causing pain and stiffness. Acid deposits can also wear off the synovial membrane and often the actual joints themselves wear down.

If you eat a balanced diet containing the correct nutrients it is possible to neutralize the excess uric acid and dissolve crystal deposits thus alleviating pain and inflammation and preventing further deterioration.

By stopping the intake of toxins and with regular exercise and a positive mind you are able, in most cases, to minimize the harmful effects of this dis-ease. The number one enemy is fast food, which contains few nutrients, but many toxic substances in the form of additives and preservatives. We have all seen the McDonalds Happy Meals kept for many years without deteriorating when even mould does not grow on them. Avoid fast food at any cost.

While I made a personal decision to walk away from mainstream allopathic medicines, I am not asking you to stop using them. It is my view that if you follow the dietary advice and exercise outlined in this book you should be able to at least reduce the amount of medications that carry a high risk of side effects causing long term damage to the internal organs.

Arthritis can also be associated with the emotions and the dis-ease can be linked to major life events such as the death of a relative, relationship breakdown, love, depression and anxiety.

Without a positive attitude no cure is available, only medication. Learn to calm the mind and find silence in meditation. "Breathe" - then the healing can begin.

Weather conditions can severely affect some people's condition, especially cold and humidity. Because of this I have chosen to settle in Mysore where we do not have cold weather or high humidity year round.

Some people will always choose to be victims of this dis-ease; that is their choice. The mind is the best medicine and you have to help yourself if you want to recover. I chose to fight and beat this dis-ease, so I can enjoy my life and later years, living a long, active and healthy life. You can do the same.

MEDICATIONS USED TO SUPPRESS ARTHRITIC CONDITIONS

The mainstream medications used to control inflammation and pain carries a high risk of side effects causing long-term damage to the internal organs.

A list of the allopathic or mainstream medicines that are commonly prescribed for arthritic conditions is included below along with their action on the body and known side effects. These drugs are mainly designed to suppress the disease or hide its symptoms and do not claim to cure. There are several side effects associated with each medication and eventually you need to start taking more medicines for the new problem caused by the old medicines and so the cycle continues.

CORTICOSTEROIDS

Prednisone and cortisone reduce inflammation and suppress the immune system.

Side effects can include: glaucoma, fluid retention, weight gain, fat deposits, high BP, behaviour and psychological effects.

DISEASE MODIFYING ANTI-RHEUMATIC DRUGS

Methotrexate and hydroxychloroquine treat the symptoms of arthritis by slowing down the immune system from attacking the joints.

Side effects can include: nausea, stomach pain, drowsiness, dizziness, blurred vision, seizures, weakness, ringing in the ears, loss of hearing, sore throat, unusual bleeding, tiredness, behaviour and psychological effects.

ANALGESICS (PAIN KILLERS)

Acetaminophen, tramadol, hydrocodone and oxycodone mask the pain but have no anti-inflammatory benefits.

Side effects can include: severe, sometimes fatal liver problems, dizziness, congestion, sore throat, drowsiness, headache, itching, constipation, loss of appetite, nausea, vomiting, weakness.

NON-STEROIDAL ANTI-INFLAMMATORY DRUGS

Ibuprofen and naproxen mask the pain and help decrease inflammation.

Side effects can include: upset stomach, mild heartburn, nausea, vomiting, bloating, dizziness, headaches, nervousness, itching, rash, ringing in your ears, increased risk of heart attacks.

For more information about drugs used to medicate arthritis see:

http://www.arthritis.org/living-with-arthritis/treatments/medication/drug-guide/

http://rheumatology.org.au/community/PatientMedicineInformation.asp

ALTERNATIVE THERAPIES FOR ARTHRITIS

From my research and experience I believe alternative therapies do work to alleviate arthritic conditions. Acupuncture, traditional Chinese medicine, naturopathy, homeopathy and other modalities all work at ridding the body of the dis-ease. Alternative therapy is not a quick fix and what works for me may not work for you and vice versa. You have to commit to a therapy, find a special healing place within it, apply a positive mind and allow the body to recover.

Alongside all therapies you must make dietary and lifestyle changes to help recovery and maintain a healthy life.

See the results of some of the evidence-based research or pilot studies on the use of yoga and other alternative therapies for arthritis on yogaclicks.com.

http://www.yogaclicks.com/YogaMeds/arthritis/4

SECTION 3: DIET AND NUTRITION FOR ARTHRITIS RELIEF AND GENERAL GOOD HEALTH

The main ingredients for your recovery are the nutritious foods and drinks that you will consume from now on.

By following the dietary guidelines from the lists below you will soon be on the road to recovery and an end to swollen, painful joints and dependency on high levels of medication.

You need to feed your body with the nutrients and vitamins it requires by eating the correct foods that are organically produced wherever possible. Too often our bodies do not absorb sufficient nutrients due to the chemicals, additives, colourings, and preservatives in our daily food, all this will change with your new diet.

Through eating a balanced and nutritious diet and the regular elimination of waste products from the body, recovery is only a few steps away.

More information about diets suitable for arthritis in general and the various kinds of arthritis can be found on the Arthritis Foundation website.

http://www.arthritis.org/living-with-arthritis/arthritis-diet/

From now on:

1. Say NO to commercially or factory pre-prepared and processed food. Generally these kinds of foods are low in nutritional value and may contain ingredients that are harmful.

2. Say YES to nutritious, fresh, whole, organically grown seasonal foods that are locally sourced wherever possible.

3. Try ingredients that are thought to affect arthritis (or gout) symptoms and see what their effect is on you. This includes both positive and negative effects. Positive effects include more flexibility and movement with less swelling and pain in your joints. Negative effects include greater stiffness, discomfort and pain.

The rest of this section gives examples of foods you should say a definite no to; foods that you can say a definite yes to; and those that are particularly important to watch out for because of their potential effect on the causal factors or symptoms of arthritis and/or gout. It also provides lists of foods according to their nutritional content (vitamins, minerals, carbohydrates, fats etc) to assist you to design a balanced diet for yourself. I find that by maintaining a balanced diet I can occasionally have something I shouldn't, because my system is not overloaded with other pollutants.

I am not going to ask anyone to be vegetarian or non-vegetarian, I think the human body can benefit from meat products especially organ meats and fish, which I include on the following lists. Some people need meat; some people don't. From a yoga point of view a vegetarian diet may make you more flexible but if you lack strength this can also be an hindrance. Studies have shown that eating animal cartilage and organ foods may be beneficial to some arthritis sufferers.

If you do choose meat, try to get organic meat from your local farm store, farmers market or the organic section at your supermarket. Too many growth hormones and antibiotics are randomly used in the commercial food chain, especially in the innocent chicken which is pumped full of antibiotics and growth hormones to meet the demands of the increasing market.

1. From now on say NO to these foods.

• Pre-packaged or canned food - especially snack foods, crackers, potato chips, cookies cakes and pizza dough. Trans fats or 'hydrogenated oils' are present in almost all processed packaged food.

• Saturated fats, usually in ice creams, full fat milk, processed cheese and meat products.

• Fried foods, french fries, potato chips, donuts, fried chicken.

• White sugar, artificial sweeteners or the simple sugars found in processed fruit juice, candy, cookies, soft drinks and some fruit yogurts.

• Refined carbohydrates, wheat and refined flour products, such as white bread, pasta, biscuits, cakes and some cereals.

- White rice or other refined grains.

- Alcohol - beer, wine and liquor.

- Cola, soft drinks, coffee, black tea.

A clear relationship between certain foods and gout has been established so if you have gout say NO to pork, prawn or crustaceans and to a degree red meat and alcohol.

Get into the habit of reading the information on packaged food to identify the contents. For example, fruit yoghurt may contain white sugar or artificial sweetener – even though it says organic and natural on the front! The packaging will also identify E numbers of chemical preservatives and colouring. As a rule of thumb the longer the list of 'things' in packaged foods the more likely it is to be a problem in terms of additives, lack of freshness and actual nutrition.

2. Say YES to many nutritious and tasty foods and drinks instead. Substitute whole foods for refined ingredients. Eat and enjoy:

- Honey, molasses, date syrup or jaggery (Indian unrefined sugar).

- Wholemeal grain cereal,

- Black rice, brown rice, natural rice and all the millet family.

- Fresh and sun dried fruit (avoid chemical dried fruits)

- Fresh vegetables cooked lightly and in salads.

- Fresh, sprouted and dried legumes (beans, peas, tofu).

- Nuts and seeds.

- Liver, organ meats and fish.

- Freshly made fruit, vegetable juices and smoothies.

- Green tea, decoctions and infusions hot and cold.

- Goat's milk, raw milk, yogurt and cottage cheese.

- Soya milk, coconut milk, almond and other nut milks.

- Olive oil (lots of it) and polyunsaturated oils.

- Ginger, garlic, spices and herbs.

Find more detail about these foods and their nutritional values later in this section.

3. Watch out for the positive or negative effects of any foods on your symptoms. A number of foods have been shown by research to have a positive or negative effect on disease symptoms including arthritis and/or gout symptoms. In addition, I have experimented with my own diet – by adding or eliminating foods I suspected were having an effect on me. I tested these effects on my symptoms over time and the following tips and lists have been assembled from a mixture of research sources alongside my own experience.

So you can make informed decisions about managing your disease through changes to your diet it is important to have knowledge about the interaction between uric acid and sodium in the body. This will also help you to understand some of the dietary and nutritional advice in this section and in Section 4 – The 14 day Diet to Restore Health

It has been shown that the build up of uric acid is a factor in the inflammation and pain associated with gout and rheumatoid arthritis.

Sodium neutralizes uric acid. When acid is produced in the body, sodium is taken from the stomach and the joints to counteract the acid. When sodium is taken from the joints calcium can be deposited, if enough sodium is present then uric acid creating calcium cannot be deposited. For more information see

http://www.arthritis.org/living-with-arthritis/tools-resources/expert-q-a/gout-questions/arthritis-or-gout.php

and

http://www.goutpal.com/810/alkaline-foods-more-myths-exposed/

It is essential to increase natural sodium in your diet. Here are some tips about how to do that and also balance the calcium and increase circulation through diet.

• Good sources of sodium rich foods are: cottage cheese, okra, cherries, strawberries, cabbage, celery, goats milk, apples, green leaves, carrot, squash, asparagus, onions, cauliflower, dried figs and prunes.

• Apple cider vinegar can dissolve acid deposits but should not be taken by people suffering from ulcers or kidney stones.

• Soya lecithin dissolves calcium deposits while cod liver oil and brewers yeast help prevent further deposits.

• Cherries, alfalfa sprouts and black currant are cleansing and help rid the body of uric acid.

• Garlic is a natural anti-inflammatory and promotes circulation.

Massaging the effected areas while taking a baking soda, Epsom salt or Radox bath can also help eliminate uric acid from the body. I find to use a soft nailbrush to massage my joints helps increase circulation.

Initially stay away from citrus fruits and nightshade (solanaceae family) vegetables such as tomatoes, peppers, aubergines and potatoes as they can be bad for arthritics. You may try them later on, after you have established your base diet, (see section 4) then you can test what their effect is on you.

If you have been diagnosed with some form of gluten intolerance (there is some evidence that the effects of gluten intolerance can exacerbate arthritis symptoms) you will need to be careful about how you include foods containing gluten in your arthritis diet. For more information on this see http://www.arthritis.org/living-with-arthritis/arthritis-diet/anti-inflammatory/gluten-free-diet.php

Foods that have been shown to be helpful in aiding recovery and the alleviation of symptoms of arthritis include:

Okra (ladies finger),	Garlic,
Figs,	Sunflower seeds,
Apple cider vinegar,	Rye,
Avocado,	Sesame seeds,
Bananas,	Papaya,
Cherries,	Turkey,
Black currants,	Walnuts,
Liver,	Ginger,
Fish especially 'oily' varieties,	Celery,
Wholemeal grains,	Millet,

Mussels,

Oysters,

Raisins,

Natural Yogurt,

Celery infusion,

Dandelion leaf infusion,

Brewers yeast,

Non-processed honey.

Foods that have been shown to be very helpful in aiding recovery and the alleviation of symptoms of gout include.

Cherries,

Berries,

Sunflower seeds,

Mustard leaves,

Green leaf vegetables e.g. spinach, bok choi. lettuce, kale

Rye,

Sesame seeds,

Millet,

Raisins,

Apple cider vinegar,

Cauliflower,

Broccoli,

Watercress,

Wheat grass,

Celery,

Garlic,

Radish,

Cabbage,

Turkey,

Walnuts,

Cherries,

Wholemeal grains,

Mussels,

Oysters,

Liver,

Fish, especially oily fish,

Oats,

Brewers yeast,

Yoghurt,

Celery infusion,

Dandelion leaf infusion.

BENEFICIAL VITAMIN, MINERAL, PROTEIN AND FAT SOURCES

In this section I list our essential nutrients and the benefits they have for our system. I then list the foods that contain the nutrients we require. Many of the foods appear several times and on different lists, showing how easy it is to choose and eat a healthy balanced diet.

VITAMINS

Vitamin A
Deficiency can cause defects in bone formation, vitamin A strengthens our immune system making us resistant to infection.

Best foods:

Spinach,

Bok choi,

Sweet potato,

Apple cider vinegar,

Carrots,

Mustard leaf,

Turnip leaf,

Beet leaf,

Kale,

Swiss chard,

Winter squash,

Broccoli,

Yoghurt,

Calf liver,

Millet,

Eggs - free range,

Bananas,

Sesame seeds,

Sunflower seeds,

Raisins,

Raw vegetables.

Vitamin B (Thiamine)
Lack of vitamin B can cause loss of muscle tone, depression, anaemia, fatigue, constipation and decreased fertility.

Best foods:

Red meat, beef heart, kidneys, liver	Soya,
Oily fish e.g. mackerel,	Crab (can be bad for Gout),
Free range eggs,	Brewers yeast.
Cheese,	

Vitamin B2 (Riboflavin)
Is beneficial to the soft tissues of the body,

Lack of Vitamin B2 can cause nervous depression, fatigue, confusion, dermatitis and eye problems.

Best foods:

Cheese,	Sesame seeds,
Almonds,	Spinach,
Red meat,	Squid,
Free range egg,	Oily fish,
Mushroom,	Raw milk.

Vitamin B5 (Pantothenic acid)
Good for liver function helps the brain and nervous system. Prevents fatigue and muscle cramps.

Best foods:

Mushrooms,	Sunflower seeds,
Cheese,	Fish,
Avocado,	Free-range chicken,
Eggs,	Liver.
Sweet potatoes	

Vitamin B6 (Pyridoxine)

Regulates red blood cell metabolism along the nervous and immune systems, lack of can lead to depression and increase risk of heart attack.

Best foods:

Sunflower seeds,	Dried prunes,
Pistachio nuts,	Bananas,
Tuna,	Avocados,
Free range chicken and turkey,	Leafy greens.

Vitamin B12 (Cobalamin)

Deficiency can lead to anaemia, fatigue and depression. Long-term deficiency can cause permanent damage to the brain and nervous system.

Best foods:

Oily fish,	All bran,
Crab,	Organic milk,
Liver,	Swiss cheese,
Tofu,	Free range eggs.

Vitamin C (Ascorbic acid)

Can be used in high doses against colds and infections and is a powerful antioxidant. The body requires it to maintain healthy blood vessels, cartilage and production of collagen.

Best foods:

Bell pepper - yellow, red, or green,	Broccoli,
Guava,	Strawberries,
Leafy vegetables,	Oranges,
Kale,	Tomato,
Kiwi fruit,	Papaya,

| Peas, | Gooseberry, |
| Grapes, | Citrus fruits. |

Vitamin D

Essential for all arthritis sufferers, as the body needs it to absorb calcium and phosphorous from foods for bone development, immune functioning and alleviation of inflammation, deficiency can increase the risk of cancer, poor hair growth and Osteomalacia.

One of the best ways of absorbing Vitamin D is sunshine.

Best foods:

Cod liver oil,	Lean pork
Oily fish,	Free range eggs,
Apple	Almond milk,
Mushrooms,	Soya milk,
Tofu,	Bananas
Caviar,	Sesame seeds
Organic milk,	Sunflower seeds.

Vitamin E

Helps prevent against heart disease, cancer and eye disease. Aids proper liver functioning and promotes radiant hair and skin.

Best foods:

Leafy vegetables,	Trout,
Spinach,	Olive oil,
Almonds,	Broccoli,
Sunflower seeds,	Squash pumpkin,
Avocado,	Kiwi fruit,
Shrimps,	Free range eggs.
Salmon,	

Vitamin F
Unsaturated fatty acids

Important in the repair and development of tissues, wound healing, hair growth and reproductive system.

Best foods:

Oils - peanut, safflower, sunflower, soy, walnut,

Nuts and seeds,

Oily fish,

Tofu,

Fresh vegetables.

Vitamin K
Essential vitamin against blood clotting can treat Osteoporosis and Alzheimer's disease and helps prevent cancer and heart disease.

Best foods:

Herbs,

Leafy vegetables, kale, spinach,

Spring onions,

Chillies,

Asparagus,

Cucumber,

Cooked soya beans,

Olive oil,

Dried fruit,

Prunes,

Blueberries,

Figs,

Tomatoes,

Egg yolk,

Liver.

Vitamin P (bioflavanoids - related to vitamin C)
Help maintain healthy blood vessels, veins and capillaries.

Best foods:

Plant based food,	Green peppers,
Citrus fruits,	Watercress.
Leafy greens, spinach,	

Notice how a lot of the same foods show up on the above lists, we do not need vitamin supplements if the food we are consuming is rich in nutrients. A lot of the same vitamins are helpful for bone and muscle health and for stopping inflammation. They are essential for arthritis sufferers.

You will also notice the same with the following list of minerals, we can eat our way to good health, enjoy all the fresh choices available, food should be enjoyed 'eat for health'.

We all react differently to certain foods, keep a diary and exclude the foods that cause any reaction, slowly add new foods so you can gauge the reaction on your system.

MINERALS

Calcium
Essential mineral for arthritis sufferers as it helps to build strong bones and teeth. It regulates muscle contractions including heartbeat.

Best foods:

Green vegetables,	Dairy products,
Seafood,	French beans,
Liver,	Tofu,
Free range eggs,	Sardines,
Farm chicken,	Pilchards.
Cheese,	

Iron
Helps the blood carry oxygen to the cells and to remove carbon dioxide.

Best foods:

Leafy greens,	Nuts,
Liver,	Dried fruit,
Free range eggs,	Whole grains,
Beans,	Brown rice.

Phosphorus
Essential for proper functioning of nerves, glands, muscles and bone formation

Best foods:

Meat,	Nuts,
Fish,	Sunflower seeds,
Free range eggs,	Broccoli,
Farm chicken,	Peas.

Magnesium
Activates enzymes.

Best foods:

Brewers yeast,	Wheat Bran,
Leafy greens,	Cocoa,
Oily fish, mackerel,	Cashews,
Almonds,	Pumpkin seeds.

Copper
Essential for bone and connective tissue production, deficiency leads to osteoporosis, joint pain and lowered immunity.

Best foods:

Seafood,	Avocados,
Leafy greens,	Goat's cheese,
Mushrooms,	Brown rice,
Seeds,	Soya,
Nuts,	Fermented tofu,
Beans pulses,	Tempeh,
Dried fruit,	Miso.

Potassium

Aids a proper digestive system, feeds the heart, kidney and muscles.

Best foods:

Leafy greens,	Oily fish,
Bananas,	Fruits,
Summer squash,	Berries,
Mushrooms,	Apple cider vinegar.
Yogurt,	

Iodine

Regulates the metabolism through the thyroid.

Best foods:

Fish,	Organic cereals and grains.
Shellfish,	

Again we see a lot of the same foods coming up.

Remember when you buy food, try to get organic or locally produced seasonal fruits, vegetables, whole grains and meat. When cooking do not use too much water and do not cook for too long, the closer to raw the more nutrients remain. DO NOT throw away any cooking water, save it and add it to your smoothies, juices or soups. Steaming is a great way to prepare fresh vegetables, no more cans or jars. Take the time and enjoy it, knowing you are actually feeding yourself to wellness.

PROTEINS

Proteins, made up mainly of amino acids, are our basic requirement, they are essential for our tissues, muscles, organs, blood and all the cells in our body.

Arthritis sufferers have to be extremely aware as protein deficiency can lead to severe attacks. Look out for early signs: lack of energy, fatigue, irregular bowel movements, constipation, swelling and increase in body weight.

Best Foods:

Muscle meat, e.g. steaks	Cottage cheese,
Kidneys, liver,	Tofu,
Farm chicken,	Soya beans,
Fish,	Seeds and nuts,
Seafood,	Green beans,
Raw milk,	Beans and legumes,
Yoghurt,	Cacao,
Farm eggs,	Sprouted beans.
Cheese,	

Essential amino acids.
Daily intake can be obtained by mixing one-part pulses with two parts brown rice or millet. It is a great carbohydrate and protein mix for your new diet.

FATS AND OILS

Most of our body's fat requirement is taken from vegetable oils and some meat, fish, cheese, nuts, seeds, raw milk and yogurt.

Sufficient fat and oil intake is essential for arthritis sufferers. We need them to lubricate our system.

Fats can have a bad image; people think if they eat fats or oils they are going to get fat but this is not necessarily the case. Our body needs fat as part of a controlled diet. High consumption of saturated fats has been shown to effect cardiac health. Likewise trans fats, often created by high cooking temperatures and deep-frying, have been linked with certain types of cancer and should be limited in the diet, so we need to be careful to use the right fats, oils and cooking methods. Cold pressed oils retain more nutrition than other oils and fats.

Best foods:

Cold pressed olive oil for salads and cooking is the best choice along with sunflower, peanut, sesame oil.

Fatty cuts of meat,

Butter, ghee, (clarified butter).

Cheese especially hard cheese,

Cream, soured cream,

Some savoury snacks and chocolate,

Coconut oil.

CARBOHYDRATES

Carbohydrates provide fuel for the body.

Best foods:

Fruits,

Sweet potato,

Quinoa,

Millet,

Beans, legumes, lentils,

Grains,

Seeds,

Oats,

Couscous,	Dairy,
Carrot,	Dried fruits,
Buckwheat,	Honey,
Brown rice,	Molasses,
Cereals,	Nuts and nut butter,
Noodles (no wheat),	Fruit juice.
Free range eggs,	

Get your carbohydrates from these natural foods that will also give you the added benefit of vitamins and minerals. Stay away from the refined over-processed carbohydrates, in cakes, ice cream, candy, jams, crisps, bread, white rice, spaghetti and most processed foods.

Our system is not designed to take on the extra burden of trying to break down these chemicals which have little or no nutritional value and are put in to food to make it last longer, look brighter, or taste sweeter.

Eating too much refined sugar, wheat, rice and other grain can lead to fatigue because the system is overloaded from refined foods blocking and over-working it.

OMEGA 3 FATTY ACIDS

Help prevent inflammation and decrease symptoms of arthritis.

Best foods:

Salmon,	Squid,
Herrings,	Flax seeds,
Sardines,	Walnuts,
Trout,	Chia seeds,
Mackerel,	Fish roe,
Oysters,	Caviar,

Soya beans,

Tofu,

Spinach,

Winter squash,

Kale,

Broccoli,

Olive oil,

Flaxseed oil,

Canola oil.

Cod liver oil.

TOP 10 RAW FOODS

We hear a lot about 'super' foods these days and sometimes what is in fashion can also carry a price tag to match. There are all types of cost effective alternatives out there, you have to learn to be your own nutritionist.

Coconut,

Chia seeds,

Leafy greens,

Seeds,

Seaweed,

Sprouts,

Blueberries,

Bee pollen,

Raw chocolate,

Cacao nibs.

TONICS AND SUPPLEMENTS

I am grateful to Dr Jag for suggesting three things that have always helped me in times of inflammation and also as a general daily health tonic. I have integrated them into the 14-day diet in the next section.

1. Apple cider vinegar that is organic and unfiltered with the natural culture 'mother of vinegar' cloudiness at the bottom and packaged in a glass container.

Take 1tbsp apple cider vinegar mixed with 1 tbsp. honey and 4 tbsp. of warm water every morning and evening at times of inflammation. At other times take the mixture once a day as a general tonic to balance uric acid in the body.

2. Instead of tea and coffee, drink hot ginger water, dandelion leaf or celery leaf infusion to help circulation and cleanse the body.

You can make your own infusions. It is easier and much cheaper than trying to find them in your local health food store. Just let the leaves dry in the sun or between a folded piece of brown paper in a cupboard, turn every 6 to 12 hours until fully dry, store in a glass container.

3. Cod liver oil capsules are still the best supplement for arthritis and should be taken daily. Cod liver oil contains beneficial omega 3 fatty acids and high amounts of vitamin A and vitamin D.

Glucosamine msm and chondroitin are both popular supplements for arthritis and both have been shown in research trials to cause no harm but have some benefits.

For more information see:

http://www.arthritis.org/living-with-arthritis/treatments/natural/supplements-herbs/glucosamine-chondroitin-osteoarthritis.php

While writing this I received an email from msn on 'How to eat your way to health'. The featured article 'The food heroes that beat health problems' shows that the world is waking up to the benefits of diet.

http://www.msn.com/en-gb/foodanddrink/quality-food-produce/the-food-heroes-that-beat-health-problems/ss-BBrtXrv?ocid=MSN_UK_NL_MO35_NO

A colleague also introduced me to the story of Seamus Mullen, a famous chef in New York, who also suffered from arthritis. His story is similar to mine. He relates how he was cured from the harmful effects of the disease with the help of a medical doctor who prescribed diet, exercise and lifestyle changes.

http://www.telegraph.co.uk/foodanddrink/11327784/Seamus-Mullen-the-chef-who-cured-himself-of-arthritis.html

http://blog.arthritis.org/stories-of-yes/seamus-mullen-rheumatoid-arthritis/

He has written a cookbook: Seamus Mullen's Hero Food: How Cooking With Delicious Things Can Make Us Feel Better (Andrew McMeel Publishing, May 2012).

SECTION 4: THE 14-DAY DIET TO RESTORE HEALTH

If you have got this far in the book, I guess you are serious enough to take the 14-day diet challenge. What have you lost if you feel no better afterwards? Believe in the challenge you are taking. Enjoy the new variations and tastes in your new diet knowing you are eating yourself back to health.

I read widely to assemble information about nutrition, diet and arthritis. Then I tried various diets myself over several years – noting the effect of the various foods on my own symptoms. From this testing the 14-day diet for arthritis relief and recovery was developed.

The diet is outlined below. In addition the restricted and non-restricted lists should be used as the basis for identifying and testing those foods that you are particularly sensitive to and may cause a flare-up of pain and stiffness.

The next section on breathing and meditation techniques compliments this diet section. I encourage you to do the exercises you can in that section, from hand exercise variations through to the Suryanamaskar sequences if possible, while at the same time modifying your diet.

The 14-day diet has 2 phases.

During Phase 1: days 1 - 4, you will establish a base diet and develop new eating habits as a template for your diet in Phase 2 over the next 10 days.

In Phase 2: days 5 - 14, you will stick to the base diet but you can play around with the recommended ingredients and gradually introduce different beneficial foods into your menu.

In both phases you are encouraged to keep a record of the effects of various foods and combinations of ingredients on your arthritis and eliminate anything you think might be having a bad effect on your symptoms. Later on you may want to re-introduce these foods to test your assumptions.

It is intended that over these 14 days you will develop the knowledge and confidence to get to the next phase - a diet tailored for you and by you that will be beneficial for the rest of your life.

Over the 14 days of the diet (except for fast day) I recommend that you take twice daily:

> 2 cod liver oil capsules or 1 tsp of cod liver oil. Cod liver oil contains beneficial omega 3 fatty acids and high amounts of vitamin A and vitamin D

> 1 tbsp of apple cider vinegar mixed with 1tbsp of honey and 4 tbsp of warm water to balance the uric acid in the body.

Do not take the cod liver oil and the apple cider vinegar mix at the same time, leave a gap of at least 30 minutes.

GOOD THINGS FOR THE TABLE

I like to keep small jars of the following on my dining table to sprinkle on my fruits, porridge, main course dishes and salads. They add nutrients and taste to my diet and they also decorate the food, remember, before we taste with the mouth we see with the eyes. Use any of the ingredients on this list to enhance your food choices during the 14-day diet.

Rock salt - not ionised for full mineral benefit,

Sunflower seeds,

Hemp seeds (ground),

Flax seeds (ground),

Sesame seeds, white & black ground or whole,

Cacao nibs,

Hemp powder,

Bee pollen,

Dried berries,

Raisins,

Toasted amaranth,

Cinnamon powder,

Honey,

Date syrup,

Nut butters - peanut, almond or cashew.

These are my choices from the many 'super' foods rich in nutrients. Find your own taste and enjoy it.

PHASE 1: DAYS 1 - 4

DAY 1

Fast for 24 hours. Eat no food. Do not worry you will not starve as you have plenty of bodily resources. Drink water when you are thirsty.

DAY 2

Begin the day with a dose of cod liver oil and the apple cider vinegar and honey mix, remembering to leave a 30-minute gap between.

Breakfast
Choice of fresh seasonal fruits sprinkled with sesame seeds, ground flax seeds and cacao nibs.

Fruit smoothie, use the same fruit so there is not too much variation.

Hot ginger water, celery leaf or dandelion leaf infusion to aid circulation.

Lunch
Mixed leaf and avocado salad, topped with sliced grapes or apple, sesame seeds and olive oil.

Fresh fruit, juice or smoothie.

Dinner
Grated carrot, beetroot, cucumber and pomegranate salad, dressed with olive oil topped with pine nuts

Raw or lightly cooked liver, or grilled or steamed fish fillet or tofu.

Fresh fruit topped with honey, sesame seeds and cacao nibs.

Bedtime
End the day with a dose of cod liver oil and the apple cider vinegar and honey mix.

Water if required.

DAY 3

Begin the day with a dose of cod liver oil and the apple cider vinegar and honey mix.

Breakfast
Fresh fruit juice,

Fresh fruit, yogurt, oats cooked or raw mixed with yogurt, honey.

Try sprinkling the fruit and oats with flax, sesame, sunflower, chia seeds, cacao nibs, or bee pollen for extra nutrients.

Do not mix too many different fruits. Remember to keep a diary to note the effects.

Hot ginger water, celery leaf or dandelion leaf infusion.

Lunch
Mixed green salad, or cooked greens dressed with olive oil and apple cider vinegar.

Millet or rice mixed with fresh corn and peas (frozen is ok)

Smoothie

Dinner
Fish poached/grilled/ baked or braised liver lightly cooked. Sweet potato roast or mash, bok choi or spinach braised with a little garlic garnished with sesame oil and seeds.

Dessert: fresh fruit.

Replace your coffee or tea habit with a healthy healing infusion or green tea.

Bedtime
End the day with a dose of cod liver oil and the apple cider vinegar and honey mix.

Water if required.

DAY 4

Begin and end the day with a dose of cod liver oil and the apple cider vinegar and honey mix.

Today keep to the same combinations of food as on the previous day, for variation cook them in a different way or choose a main ingredient that is different to your Day 3 choice. This will help you better assess any reactions.

Breakfast
Fresh fruit juice, fresh fruit, yogurt, oats cooked or raw mixed into the yogurt, honey.

Try sprinkling the fruit and oats with seeds, flax, sesame, and sunflower for extra nutrients.

Celery leaf or dandelion leaf infusion.

Lunch
Raw salad, or cooked greens, dressed with olive oil and apple cider vinegar.

Millet or rice mixed with fresh corn or peas (frozen is ok)

Smoothie

Dinner
Fish poached/grilled/ baked or braised liver. Sweet potato roast or mash, bok choi or spinach braised with a little garlic garnished with sesame oil and seed.

Dessert: fresh fruit.

Bedtime

Apple cider vinegar and honey in hot water.

Cod liver oil

Water if required.

In the following days you can gradually start adding from the lists of foods that have been shown to be beneficial for arthritis in Section 3. Remember to maintain your same base foods.

Replace your coffee or tea habit with a healthy healing infusion or green tea.

Over these first 4 days you have set up a diet that restricts the foods you eat to those that are nutritious and beneficial for arthritis. These 4 days are the template (or base diet) that you can use for the next 10 days. If you require more meat protein, add it to your lunch plan.

PHASE 2: DAYS 5 - 14

Now stick with that Day 1 – 4 base diet for the next 10 days. You may choose to have fast days on day 5 and day 10. If you feel you want to add more items from the YES' list in Section 3 do so gradually and keep a diary of what you are eating and what you are adding, noting their effects on your symptoms. For variety, try cooking ingredients in different ways, steaming, baking etc and experiment with adding various items from the 'Good things for the table list' to your dishes.

PHASE 3: DAY 15 - FOREVER

By now you will have a clearer idea about the foods you enjoy that do not exacerbate your arthritis symptoms. You will also have practiced keeping track of the impact of diet on your symptoms and general health. From here on you can design your own diets and eating patterns and enjoy a wide range of foods that are good for you. If my theory is correct you will have come some way along the path to curing your arthritis, and reducing the associated inflammation and pain.

SECTION 5: BASIC ASHTANGA YOGA FOR ARTHRITIS RELIEF

YOGA AND ARTHRITIS

"Yoga can ease movement, improve posture, and align bones. A regular practice can create space and ease pain in damaged joints, and help to prevent the cartilage erosion that causes the pain of arthritis.

It can also be a good way to build muscle strength (for example hand grip) because, practised correctly, it doesn't put too much pressure on the joints – provided you don't overdo it when joints are flaring.

Yoga, meditation, mindfulness, and pranayama (breathing techniques), can also help you mentally deal with the pain and improve your sense of wellbeing helping to reduce the stress and tension caused by the discomfort and pain of arthritis. This, in turn, can promote better sleep and relaxation, helping to improve all-round physical health, wellbeing and vitality."

This quote is from the YogaClicks website which has a section about how yoga can help ease the symptoms of arthritis. It also has information about a number of clinical studies on the topic that support the quote. Sign up with YogaClicks to learn more.

http://www.yogaclicks.com/YogaMeds/arthritis/4

While any yoga practice can benefit your health and ease the symptoms of various arthritic conditions I have concluded from my own experience that Ashtanga yoga has the most to offer me. Ashtanga yoga translated is 8 limbs of yoga, it is also a name given to a particular series of yoga but all yoga asana practice is Hatha yoga.

Ashtanga yoga as we know it today comes from the Yoga Korunta, an ancient manuscript discovered by T Krishnamacharya in the National Archives of India in Calcutta. The text is said to contain lists of different asana groupings as well as teachings on vinyasa, dristhi, bandha and mudra.

T Krishnamacharya is regarded as one of the most influential yoga teachers of the 20th century and can be credited with the revival of hatha yoga in India.

The ashtanga yoga series is considered to be a complete series for a healthy body and mind. The techniques involved have the capacity to rid the body of dis-ease through purification.

Ashtanga yoga began spreading in the late1960s and early 70s after the early foreigners from America and Europe came to practice it with Pattabhi Jois in Mysore. In the 1980s when celebrities like Madonna, Sting, and Paul Simon started the practice, ashtanga started spreading to most cities worldwide.

You can find out more about ashtanga yoga and the K Pattabhi Jois Ashtanga Yoga Institute here http://kpjayi.org

I practice traditional ashtanga yoga. However, I will first provide you with a modified version designed for beginners who have rheumatoid arthritis and/or gout.

Over time I hope you will work your way through the series and maintain a regular practice, eating the correct foods and living a life free of debilitating pain.

While moving the joints can be painful; not moving the joints destroys them. Incorrect movement damages joints; while correct movement heals.

Some critics of ashtanga yoga say that the practice is too strong, that women become like men physically, that many people get injured and that you have to be a young gymnast to do it. I have already mentioned earlier, it is not ashtanga that breaks bodies it is ones own ego that does the breaking. Always practice within your own ability and respect your body to prevent unnecessary injuries.

Pattabi Jois used to say, "everyone can practice ashtanga yoga but a lazy person".

Practice within your own limitations. Gradually go forward adding new asanas when you are ready, but most of all practice with awareness. Ashtanga encourages you to learn about your own body and how it works.

Ashtanga has 4 main principles:

- Bandha, (body locks)
- Ujayi breath (breathing with sound),
- Dristhi, (gazing point).
- Vinyasa, (breathing and movement)

When we bring these elements together we practice meditation in movement.

Ashtanga yoga represents the eight limbs of yoga, of which asana (posture) is number three. Asana or posture is the limb of yoga that represents the exercises in this section.

A description of eight limbs follows so you can see where asana fits within a broader yogic way of living.

1. Yama: the five external moral restraints.

Ahimsa – non-violence.

Sathya – truthful/ non lying.

Bramacharya – control of sexual desires.

Asthya – no stealing/ jealousy.

Aparigraha – non-possessiveness, freedom from desire.

2. Niyama: the five internal observances, self discipline.

Saucha – cleanliness, purity.

Santosha – contentment.

Tapas - austerity, self discipline.

Swadhya – self-study and of sacred texts.

Ishwara – worship of the supreme.

3. Asana – posture.

4. Pranayama – breath control/ vital energy.

5. Prathyahara – turning inward, withdrawal of the senses.

6. Dharana – concentration calming the distractions of the mind.

7. Dhyana - meditation, awareness without focus.

8. Samadhi – spiritual enlightenment.

Now, I will outline the main principles of ashtanga so that you can understand them and learn how to use them to improve your mobility and general health.

Even if your condition is so bad that you can only start with the hand exercise, learn how to use the three bandhas and ujayi breath and to do each exercise with awareness and mindfulness.

In ashtanga yoga, bandha helps us separate the top half and the bottom half of the body so we can work them independently, making the body light and strengthening the internal core. Try to keep bandha awareness throughout your yoga practice and link with your breathing even if you are only doing the hand exercises.

BANDHA (BODY LOCKS)

The three bandhas used in ashtanga yoga are:

- Moola bandha – situated around the perineum/pelvic floor.
- Udiyana bandha – 2 inch or 3 fingers width below the naval.
- Jalandhara bandha – in the throat region.

MOOLA BANDHA: THE ROOT LOCK

To find moola bandha:

- Sit on the floor in a padmasana or half lotus position.
- Feel the sitting bones, draw them together towards the centre then relax the buttocks without releasing the sitting bones.
- Now focus on the pubic and tail bone and bring them together into the centre
- Moola bandha is where these 4 points meet, draw the energy up from that point

To find moola bandha another way try this version, (thanks to David Svenson for this description).

Imagine you are out and about and you suddenly feel the urge to go for a 'pee' a number 1. You would consciously tighten the muscles in the pubic area, which would stop you releasing.

Now imagine the same situation and you need to go for a 'poo' a number 2. Again you would tighten the muscles, this time at the rear and stop the release.

So, in between number 1 and number 2 is number 1½. This is the point where moola bandha is located. Now draw up the energy from that point, this is moola bandha.

UDDIYANA BANDHA- ABDOMINAL LOCK

Uddiyana bandha is situated 3 finger widths below the naval. Draw in at this point and hold, linking with the top of moola bandha whilst maintaining inhalation and exhalation. With practice when you draw in udiyana bandha, moola bandha will automatically engage.

Pattabi Jois used to say, 'hold moola bandha and uddiyana at all times, not just in your asana practice.' This means whenever you are walking, driving or sitting. When practiced consistently it will make your internal core strong, prevent urinary and intestine problems and protect the lower back.

JALANDHARA BANDHA - CHIN LOCK

Jalandhara bandha is situated in the throat region; whereas moola bandha seals the bottom of an imaginary tube. Jalandhara bandha seals the top.

To find jalandhara bandha

• Sit with moola bandha and udiyana bandha engaged, with a straight back and shoulders squared.

• Lengthen your cervical spine then drop the chin slightly, this is jalandhara bandha.

Do not just bend your chin and let your shoulders sink forward.

Jalandhar bandha is not engaged in all asanas like the other two bandhas. It is used only in certain asanas.

UJAYI BREATH (BREATHING WITH SOUND)

Ujayi breath is simply breathing with sound (it is not the same as ujayi pranayama).

• Stand tall or sit in half lotus position with a straight back, moola bandha and uddiyana bandha engaged.

• Close your eyes and exhale with the mouth open making the sound ahhhhhhh.

• Feel where the sound is coming from; you should feel a small vibration in the glottis (lower throat).

• Now repeat the same exercise with the mouth closed. The vibration and the internal sound is increased and more pronounced in the glottis, almost like a elongated sigh. Feel the length of the breath.

You should only hear the sound on the exhalation. It can be a soft noise that you alone can hear or stronger where other people can also hear. Both are correct as long as you feel the vibration.

Try to create a rhythm with the breath and stay with it throughout the practice - like a mantra to focus awareness

The ashtanga yoga primary series was created to burn the accumulated toxins from the body. With regular practice of vinyasa, bandha and ujayi breath you create an internal fire burning up accumulated toxins from the body

All breathing should be done with the nose not the mouth.

DRISTHI (GAZING POINT)

Dristhi is the gazing point within the asana. It holds the attention, improves concentration and brings about a feeling of oneness, resulting in meditation in movement. There are different Dristhi used in different asanas.

Urdhva dristhi – up to space

Brumadhya dristhi – third eye (middle of forehead)

Nasarga dristhi - tip of the nose

Parsva dristhi - left side or right side

Nabhi dristhi - navel

Hastagra dristhi - tip of middle finger

Angusta dristhi - tip of the thumb

Padagra dristhi - tip of big toe

VINYASA

Vinyasa refers to the movement and breath within the sequence of the asana,

As the sage Vamana says, 'Vina vinyasa yogena asanadin na karayet (O yogi, do not do asana without vinyasa).'

G. Mohan succinctly explains the modern meaning of *vinyāsa* in his biography of his teacher T. Krishnamacharya, (who was also the teacher of Sri K. Pattabhi Jois):

"A special feature of the asana system of Krishnamacharya was vinyasa. Many yoga students today are no doubt familiar with this word – it is increasingly used now, often to describe the 'style' of a yoga class, as in 'hatha vinyasa' or 'vinyasa flow'. Vinyasa is essential, and probably unique, to Krishnamacharya's teachings. As far as I know, he was the first yoga master in the last century to introduce this idea. A vinyasa, in essence, consists of moving from one asana, or body position, to another, combining breathing with the movement."

To complete this section I will now outline a series of basic exercises for improving your breathing and opening your chest. I then outline a couple of meditation techniques.

Finally, I outline a series of basic exercises to help you regain or increase your mobility. You will then be well prepared to move onto the Ashtanga Yoga Primary Series in Section 6.

BREATHING EXERCISES

Ten reasons why breathing exercises are beneficial:

1. Improve brain function

2. Soothe the nervous system

3. Clean the lungs

4. Calm the mind

5. Enhance relaxation

6. Improve sleep

7. Boost energy

8. Enhance rest

9. Merge the left and right side of the brain

10. Prepare the mind and body for meditation.

Following are a set of five breathing exercises that, if practiced daily they will help you gain the benefits listed above and prepare you for the ashtanga practice in Section 6. The left nostril is generally associated with 'calming' and the 'feeling' right side of the brain, while the right nostril is associated with 'energy' and the 'thinking' left side of the brain. Alternating your breathing through both nostrils activates the whole brain.

BREATHING EXERCISE 1. INCREASING LUNG CAPACITY

Sit in a comfortable position with legs crossed or kneeling, back straight, engage moola bandha and uddiyana bandha.

1. Inhale for a silent count of 4; exhale for a silent count of 4

2. Inhale for 5; exhale for 5

3. Inhale for 6; exhale for 6

4. Inhale for 7; exhale for 7

5. Inhale for 8; exhale for 8

6. Inhale for 7; exhale for 7

7. Inhale for 6; exhale for 6

8. Inhale for 5; exhale for 5

9. Inhale for 4; exhale for 4.

If you cannot initially inhale for 7 or 8 counts, do the exercise for 6 counts. With a few days of practice your lungs will become more elastic and you can build to 7 and 8 breaths, Maximum inhalation should be a silent count of 10.

If it feels good do it again with full awareness. Feel the inhalation expand the lungs, bringing the new life force and then the exhalation taking away the waste, cleansing the whole system.

BREATHING EXERCISE 2. BREATHING WITH AWARENESS

Once you have increased your lung capacity you can move on to a breathing technique that takes some practice to perfect. It consists of an even long inhalation followed by an even long exhalation whilst maintaining awareness of each breath. Imagine you are breathing up and down a tube.

1. Sit in a comfortable position with legs crossed and back straight, engage moola bandha and uddiyana bandha.

2. Inhale evenly for a silent count of 8. Watch the breath as it fills up from the base of your lungs, passing the stomach (no stomach breathing) high into the chest to the top of the lungs, you can feel your lungs rise in the dip between your collarbones.

3. Exhale evenly for a silent count of 8, controlling the release. Feel the breath expel waste air completely from the base of the lungs.

Repeat steps 2 and 3 five times.

Over time you can gradually increase the count of each breath (maximum 15), increasing the count only when you are ready.

BREATHING EXERCISE 3. ALTERNATE NOSTRIL BREATHING,

1. Sit in a comfortable position with legs crossed and back straight, engage moola bandha and uddiyana bandha.

2. Make a hand mudra with right hand (as shown in photo), close the right nostril with the thumb and inhale through the left nostril for a count of 8.

3. Close left nostril with ring finger and exhale through the right nostril for silent count of 8.

4. Keep the left nostril closed with ring finger and inhale through right nostril to the count of 8.

5. Close the right nostril with the thumb and exhale through the left nostril for silent count of 8.

Repeat steps 2 to 5 (1 round) five times. Gradually increase the number of rounds when you feel ready (maximum of 20 rounds).

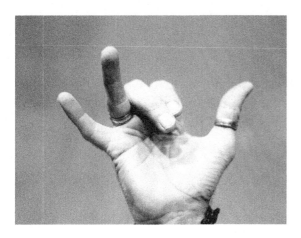
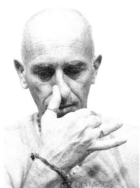
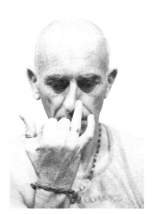

BREATHING EXERCISE 4. NADI SHODHANA

Nadi Shodhana is a nerve cleansing pranayama

    1. Sit in a comfortable position with legs crossed and back straight, engage moola bandha and uddiyana bandha.

    2. Make a hand mudra with the right hand, close the right nostril with the thumb of the right hand; exhale from the left nostril for 8 silent counts

    3. Inhale for only 4 counts through the same left nostril

    4. Close left nostril with ring finger, exhale from the right nostril for 8 counts

    5. Inhale for 4 counts through the right nostril

    6. Close the right nostril with the thumb; exhale for 8 counts from left nostril.

Repeat steps 2 to 6 (1 round) five times. Gradually increase the number of rounds when you feel ready (maximum of 20 rounds).

If you cannot exhale to the count of 8 do 6 exhalation and 4 inhalation. With practice your lungs will get stronger and you will be able do the full count of 8 or more.

In this exercise, remember to exhale for twice the length of the inhalation.

This technique can be used at the end of your yoga practice or any time you feel tension or pain throughout the day.

If you concentrate on the breath when you are feeling pain, it will cloud the pain. Through correct breathing techniques with awareness you can close pain gateways. BKS Iyengar said: "The mind is the controller of the body but the breath is the controller of the mind".

BREATHING EXERCISE 5. CHEST OPENING

1. Sit on the floor legs straight, take the hands back 30cm, fingers facing forwards.

2. Inhale, breathing into the top of the lungs, lifting and opening the chest, head back.

3. Exhale, keeping the chest open and high.

Repeat steps 2 and 3 seven times. Each time you repeat step 2 open the chest a little more.

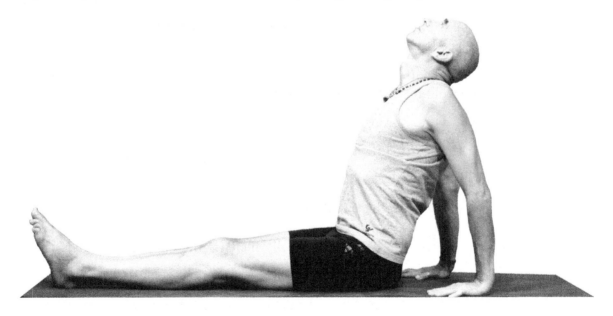

MEDITATION

There are many meditation techniques. I will explain only two very simple yet powerful ones that I find useful for relieving stress and to bring a sense of calm.

The first one can be practiced anywhere: sitting at home, waiting in the car, on the bus, anywhere when you have a few minutes and you want a quick clearing of the senses and a calm mind. Once learned this valuable tool will help silence the mind.

MEDIATION TECHNIQUE 1

1. Sit in any comfortable position preferably with legs crossed, back straight and eyes closed.

2. Engage mula, udiyana, and jalandhara bandha.

3. Inhale slowly filling your lungs keeping full awareness of the breath.

4. Exhale slowly until your lungs feel empty maintaining full awareness of the breath.

Try to tune into your breath, feel the air passing through your nostrils when inhaling and exhaling, maintain that awareness. When you lose attention bring it back by concentrating on your breath. As you progress you will be able to hold the 'silence' for longer periods without losing attention.

In the beginning try meditating using this technique for 5 minutes 3 times each day. Then you can gradually increase your mediation sessions to 15-minute sittings two or three times each day.

Instead of closing your eyes you may keep them open and concentrated on a single point, for example, the flame of a candle, a light or the centre of a flower. If you use this variation try not to blink. Your eyes may start to water but maintain awareness of the point of concentration

MEDITATION TECHNIQUE 2

If you are having problems sleeping or relaxing because of worrying thoughts, try this technique to shift awareness from the mind to the body.

1. Lay down on the floor or a bed in supine position, close your eyes and become aware of your breath through slow relaxed breathing.

2. Imagine a blue coloured sheet of fabric slowly starting to cover your body, starting at the toes and slowly coming up the body until finally it covers your whole body including the head.

Do not rush this exercise; it should take around 10 minutes for the imaginary blue cloth to cover the whole body. By then you should have shifted your awareness from the mind to the body, experiencing full awareness of the body. Relax there with a quiet mind.

If necessary the exercise can be repeated.

EXERCISES TO REGAIN MOBILITY

Depending on your condition a lot of pain can generally be felt in the hands. The hands are essential in your yoga practice as you 'ground' with the hands and the feet, as in urdva mukhasana (downward facing dog). So you need to get the hands and fingers working again.

If you follow the dietary advice (in section 3) to rid yourself of pain and swelling, massage your joints with oil and follow these simple exercises the muscles and tendons of the hands will start to become strong again.

Before you start any exercises, and to get the most out of them, you will need to prepare your joints with massage or manipulation. The first few exercise below are about massaging and strengthening the fingers. Find more information on the general benefits of massage for arthritis here

http://www.arthritis.org/living-with-arthritis/treatments/natural/other-therapies/massage/massage-benefits.php

I generally use rosemary or ginger oil when I am preparing my joints. You can also use alternatives from the list of essential oils below.

Essential oils have a beneficial effect when massaged into the skin. Always test a small amount of oil first to make sure you have no allergic reaction, if you do have a reaction you can add a base oil (coconut, vegetable or olive) to the essential oil to dilute it, or simply try another essential oil.

Rosemary oil - promotes circulation.

Camphor oil - diuretic for arthritis and gout

Ginger oil - beneficial against rheumatism, calcification of joints and muscle pain

Peppermint oil - reduces pain and inflammation.

Juniper oil - diuretic

Marjoram oil – eases stiff painful joints

Cayenne pepper oil - relieves muscle and joint pain.

Chamomile oil - stimulates circulation and detoxifies the blood.

If you choose this type of yoga-based therapy you have to start with a positive mind, re-learn to use your hands and work against the deterioration that is taking place. The muscles and tendons are strengthened through these simple exercises, helping to support weak joints and restore mobility and strength.

All the following exercises should be done with full awareness, feeling the sensation, allow each exercise to feel like a meditation.

HAND EXERCISE 1

Apply a couple of drops of oil to the knuckle and finger joints of the right hand and massage it in.

Massage each knuckle by rotating the joint, hold the finger at the first joint and rotate the knuckle joint, first clockwise then anticlockwise, do not forget the base of the thumb.

Then continue massaging from the web of the finger down the length of the finger, paying special attention to the finger joints and the fingertips.

Repeat on left hand.

When you have completed both hands, drop some oil on the wrists and do the same clock-wise and anticlockwise rotations.

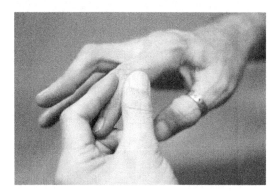

HAND EXERCISE 2

Hold the right hand upright in front of the chest.

Bend fingers from the knuckles to 90 degrees, keeping the fingers straight

Repeat ten times.

Repeat with left hand.

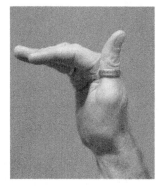

HAND EXERCISE 3

With your hand in the same position bend from the first finger joints to 90 degrees.

You may notice the fingers do not bend in unison, so you can bend each finger and thumb individually, you can help the joint to bend by supporting it with the fingers of the other hand

Do not apply too much force, only work to the edge of discomfort not into it.

The above techniques can also be modified for the feet and ankles.

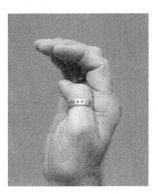

HAND EXERCISE 4

Stand at a desk, kitchen counter or kneel on your yoga mat.

Place your hands down on the surface with fingers spread, remembering only to go to your barrier of discomfort. It is essential to breathe with awareness and engage moola and udiyana bandha.

Stretch out the fingers on exhalation, again inhale, exhale and stretch out the fingers a little more tune in to the feeling in your hands.

Next on each exhale push down individually with each fingertip. Repeat with all fingers and thumb.

Next push down at each of the finger joints.

Then push down at each knuckle.

Then push down between the thumb and the first finger.

Then feel the pads of the hands where they meet the surface.

Keep you wrist independent so the pressure is in your hands.

Change hands and repeat

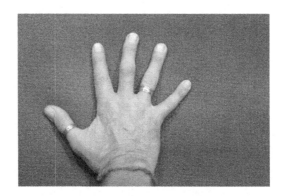

Repeat five to ten times with each hand with awareness on your breath.

Another variation of this exercise is to massage oil into both hands, bring the hands together in prayer position then spread the fingers, keeping both hands touching, individually press the finger tips together, then the finger joints, the knuckles, the palms. Release your hands, make a fist with each hand and then relax them, Open again on the exhale and repeat.

These exercises will give you a strong foundation for your Suryanamaskar practice.

Note: moola bandha and udiyana bandha should be engaged throughout the whole practice. If you find you have released the bandhas re-engage them.

Breathe with sound 'ujayi breath' with an even inhalation and exhalation.

ARM EXERCISE

While in the same position as Hand exercise 4, make sure it is the hands not the wrists that are supporting your arms. Now check the eyes of the elbows. They should be facing each other. If not, try to align them, this could feel strange at first but it can be corrected and realigned. While you do this, make sure you do not close your shoulders. The shoulders and chest should be open with the scapula drawn down the back.

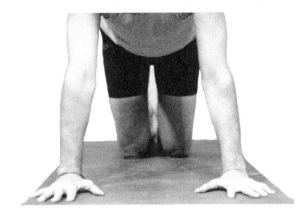 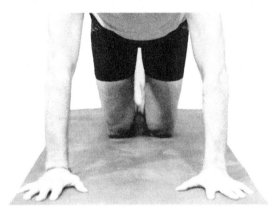

HANDS AND SHOULDERS EXERCISE

1. Kneel on the floor with hands on the ground, set your foundation.

2. Bring your shoulders above your hands, check the eyes of the elbows are facing each other.

3. Exhale, slowly lower yourself down, elbows in down to chaturanga (plank) position.

4. Inhale come back up, maintain full awareness.

Repeat five to ten times.

Remember it is better to build up strength slowly, respecting your body. This is not a quick fix; it is the first step to regaining your strength and flexibility.

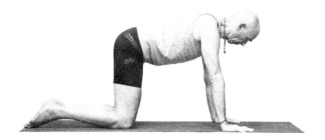

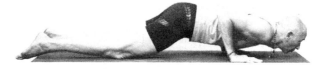

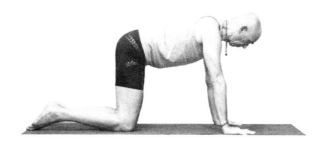

HANDS, SHOULDERS, LOWER BACK AND CHEST EXERCISE

1. Kneel on the floor with hands on the ground, set your foundation. Bring your shoulders above your hands, checking the 'eyes' of the elbows.

2. Exhale, slowly lowering down with elbows in to chaturanga, plank position.

3. Inhale, raise the chest, arching the lower back, firm foundation in the hands open chest and shoulders, coming up into urdhva mukha/upward facing dog.

4. Exhale, bringing the hips back to child pose, take 5 full breaths.

Repeat five to ten times, with awareness.

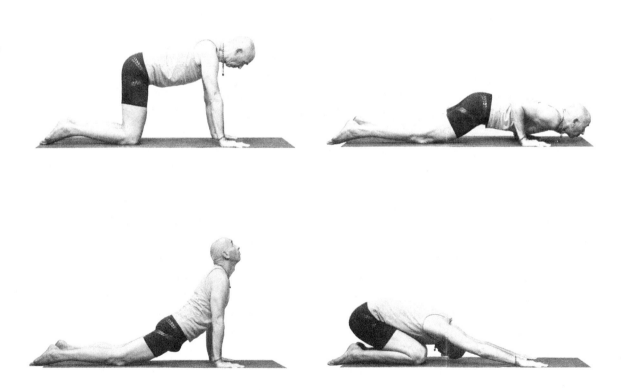

FEET EXERCISES

The exercises for the hands can be modified for the feet. Apply an essential oil first to help increase the circulation.

In acupuncture the feet are very important because this is where many of the meridians end or start. The soles of the feet have points that represent the internal organs, the kidney point is situated at the bridge of the foot towards the centre of the sole, massage this area to stimulate the kidneys and help cleansing.

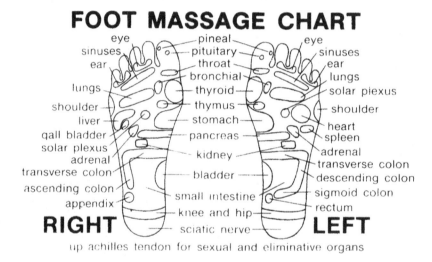

FOOT MASSAGE CHART

The above exercises are good for the whole body as they bring body awareness that will be beneficial for the asana practice, where you 'feel' the ground and learn a firm foundation.

Once your limbs and joints are loosened up and more mobile you are ready for the next level of exercise. The ashtanga yoga primary series is outlined in the next section.

When you are ready start Suryanamaskar. The instructions are in the next section. Do Suryanamaskar A initially and work towards Suryanamaskar B. Maintaining bandha and breath awareness.

When you can do ten Suryanamaskar A, change to 5 Suryanamaskar A then 3 Suryana-maskar B. increasing to 9 Suryanamaskar A and 5 Suryanamaskar B with bandha and breath awareness.

When you can complete this many rounds of Suryanamaskar A & B comfortably you are ready to move on to the Standing asana series in the next section.

If you are happy doing just the suryanamaskar continue and add more rounds as you build strength, Challenge yourself to complete 27 then 54 then 108 rounds of Suryanamaskar when practicing with full awareness on bandha and breath.

Regular practice of Suryanamaskar alone can give many benefits to the practitioner.

SECTION 6: ASHTANGA YOGA PRIMARY SERIES

In this section both numerical symbols (e.g. 1) and Sanskrit words for numbers (e.g. ekam =1, dwe = 2 etc) are used. In some asanas (such as Padangusthasana – Big toe pose the numerical symbol does not align with the corresponding Sanskrit number because the first movement is done in preparation for the sequence of the asana.

In others such as sitting asanas the last Sanskrit number ending vinyasa then continues back to Sapta jump through the 7th vinyasa movement to start the new asana because over time the vinyasa count has changed since Pattabhi Jois first started teaching, originally practitioners would come back to standing and each new asana would start at ekam

In Mysore style led classes the teacher calls the Sanskrit numbers and students change position (with vinyasa) as described below.

This is the sequence of ashtanga Sanskrit count as taught by Sharath Jois at KPJAYI Mysore in 2016.

OPENING MANTRA

Om
Vande gurunam caranaravinde, sandarsita svatma sukhava bodhe.
Nih sreyase jangalikayamane samasara hala hala mohasantyai.

Abahu purusakaram sankhacakrasi dharinam.
Sahasra sirasam svetam pranamami patanjalim

Translation

I bow to the lotus feet of the Gurus.
The awakening happiness of ones own self revealed,
Beyond better, acting like the jungle physician,
Pacifying delusion, the poison of samsara.

Taking the form of a man to the shoulders,
Holding a conch, a discus and a sword,
One thousand heads white,
To Patanjali, I salute

SURYANAMASKAR A – SALUTE TO THE SUN

1. Ekam inhale – raise the arms and stretch tall lifting from the elbows extending the armpits and side trunk. This will allow the tissue to extend making binds easier later in the practice.

2. Dwe exhale – fold forward from the hips extending the hands to the floor.

3. Trini inhale – head up only.

4. Chatwari exhale – jump or walk back into chaturanga, plank position.

5. Pancha inhale – raise the chest, look up (upward facing dog), try to lift the thighs from the floor with feet flat and pointing back, push the pelvis down extending the lower back from the sacrum, lifting the chest, (this is the first backbend) open the shoulders bringing the shoulder blades (scapula) down the back releasing the tension.

6. Shat exhale - raise the hips (downward facing dog), lift the tail bone, push back with the upper thighs draw in uddiyana bandha, looking towards the naval, nabhi dristhi, take 5 breaths with sound.

7. Sapta inhale - jump forward, head up.

8. Hastu exhale - head down.

9. Nava inhale - stretch tall, raise both arms lifting from the elbows, looking towards the thumbs.

Samasthiti - Release, bring the hands down, stand tall.

Repeat the whole sequence Suryanamaskar five times.

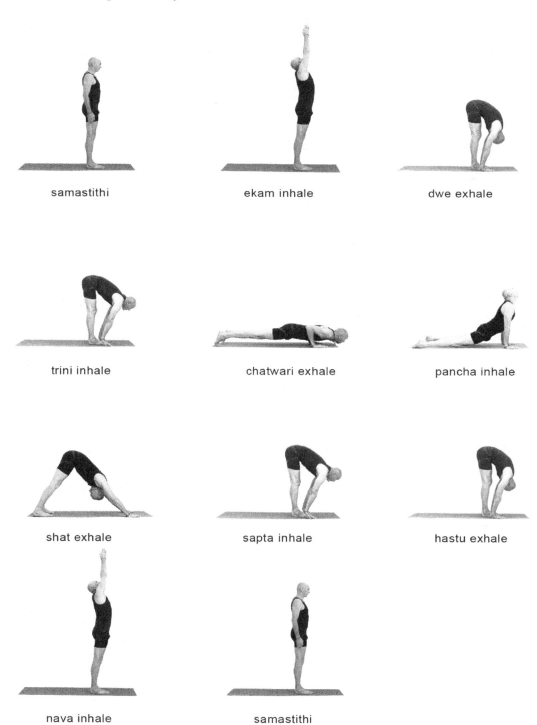

samastithi

ekam inhale

dwe exhale

trini inhale

chatwari exhale

pancha inhale

shat exhale

sapta inhale

hastu exhale

nava inhale

samastithi

MODIFICATIONS

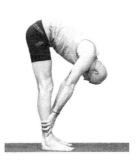

2. Dwe exhale fold forward from the hips, catch the calves or ankles.

4. Chatwari exhale walk back, lower the knees to the floor, bring shoulders over the hands, lower down to plank position, building strength in the shoulder girdle. Take an extra breath if required when going down.

7. Sapta inhale walk forward to 2nd position, head up.

SURYANAMASKAR B

1. Ekam inhale – bend the knees, stretch tall raising both arms lifting from the elbows looking towards the thumbs.

2. Dwe exhale – fold forward from the hips extending the hands to the floor.

3. Trini inhale – head up only.

4. Chatwari exhale – jump or walk back into chaturanga, plank position.

5. Pancha inhale – raise the chest, look up (upward facing dog), try to lift the thighs from the floor with feet flat pointing back, push the pelvis down extending the lower back from the sacrum, lifting the chest, open the shoulders bringing the scapula down the back releasing the tension.

6. Shat exhale – raise the hips, (downward facing dog).

7. Sapta inhale – right foot forward, back foot at 45 degrees heel down, pushing the outside of the back foot into the ground, turning the thigh inwards. Right heel should be in line with the middle of the arch of left foot. Shoulders square, raise the arms lifting from the elbows, hands together, looking up towards the thumbs.

8. Hastu exhale – all the way down into chaturanga, plank position.

9. Nava inhale - raise the chest, look up (upward facing dog), try to lift the thighs from the floor with feet flat pointing back, push the pelvis down extending the lower back from the sacrum, lifting the chest open the shoulders, bringing the scapula down the back releasing the tension.

10. Dasa exhale – Raise the hips (downward facing dog).

11. Eka dasa inhale - left foot forward, back foot 45 degrees heel down, pushing the outside of the back foot into the ground, turning the thigh inwards. Left heel should be in line with the middle of the arch of right foot. Shoulders square, raise the arms lifting from the elbows, hands together looking up towards the thumbs.

12. Dwe dasa exhale - all the way down into chaturanga, plank position

13. Trio dasa inhale - raise the chest, look up (upward facing dog), try to lift the thighs from the floor with feet flat pointing back, push the pelvis down extending the lower back from the sacrum, lifting the chest, open the shoulders, bringing the scapula down the back releasing the tension.

14. Chatur dasa exhale - raise the hips (downward facing dog), lift the tail bone push back with the upper thighs draw in udiyana bandha, looking towards the naval, Nabhi dristhi, 5 breaths with sound.

15. Pancha dasa inhale – jump forward head up.

16. Sho dasa exhale – head down.

17. Sapta dasa inhale – bend the knees, stretch tall, raise both arms lifting from the elbows, hands together, looking at the thumbs.

Samasthiti - Release, bring the hands down, stand tall.

Repeat the whole sequence Suryanamaskar B three times.

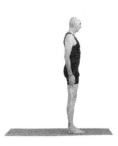

samastithi

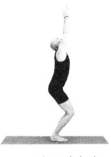

ekam inhale

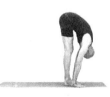

dwe exhale

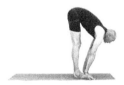

trini inhale

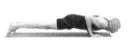

chatwari exhale

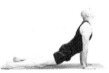

pancha inhale

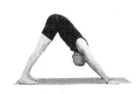

shat exhale

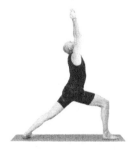

sapta inhale

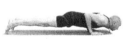

hastu exhale

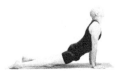

nava inhale

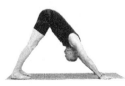

dasa exhale

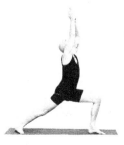

eka dasa inhale

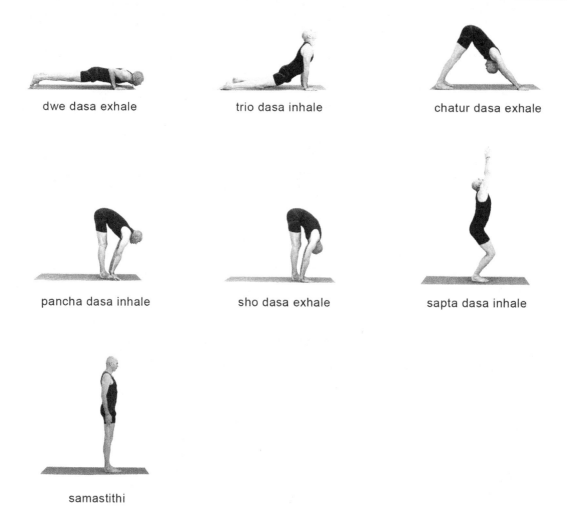

dwe dasa exhale

trio dasa inhale

chatur dasa exhale

pancha dasa inhale

sho dasa exhale

sapta dasa inhale

samastithi

MODIFICATIONS

4. Chatwari exhale - walk back, lower the knees, bring shoulders over the hands lower down, building strength in the shoulder girdle. Take an extra breath going down if required.

7. Sapta inhale - right foot forward raise the arms, take an extra breath if required.

8. Hastu exhale - drop the knees lower down with the shoulders. Take an extra breath if required. Repeat same technique left side.

STANDING SERIES OF ASANAS

PADANGUSTHASANA – FOOT BIG TOE POSE

1. Jump the feet hip distance apart, hands on waist.

2. Ekam inhale - catch the big toes, head up.

3. Dwe exhale - fold forward extending the crown of the head to the floor. Straight legs, bring the weight forward more into the toes increasing the hamstring stretch, raise the tailbone. Open elbows out to the side opening the chest. Take 5 breaths with sound. Dhristi nose.

4. Trini inhale- head up only, exhale

Continue to next asana.

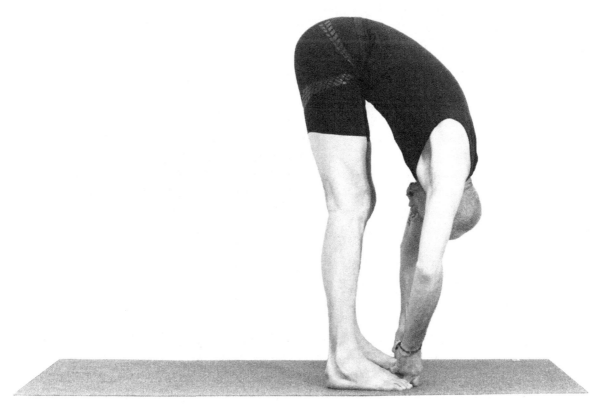

Padangusthasana

MODIFICATION

If you can't catch your toes catch your calves or ankles and bend your knees slightly.

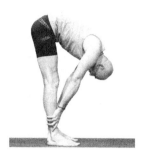

PADAHASTASANA – HANDS TO FEET POSE

1. Ekam inhale – place the hands under the feet, palms facing upwards.

2. Dwe exhale - fold forward extending the crown of the head to the floor. Straight legs, bring the weight forward more into the toes increasing the hamstring stretch, raise the tailbone. Open elbows out to the side opening the chest. Take 5 breaths with sound. Dhristi nose.

3. Trini inhale – head up only, exhale there.

4. Inhale - hands on waist come to standing position.

5. Exhale Samasthiti - jump the feet back together, release the hands stand tall.

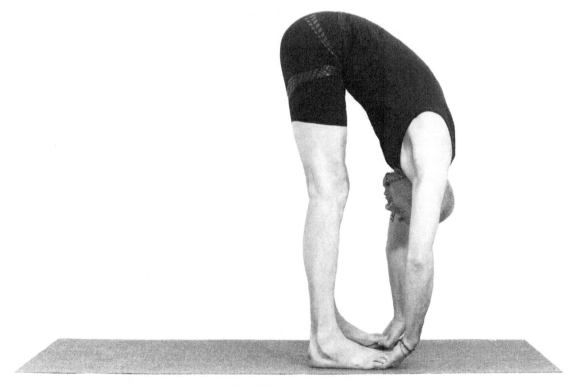

Padahastasana

MODIFICATION

If you can't place the hands underneath the toes, catch your calves or ankles and bend your knees slightly

UTTHITA TRIKONASANA A – EXTENDED TRIANGLE POSE

1. Ekam inhale – jump or step the right foot to the right hand-side, arms out stretched, feet should be around 3 ft apart, or same length as your leg, right foot pointing forward back foot 45 degrees, right heel should be in line with the middle of the arch of the left foot

2. Dwe exhale – looking into the middle finger of the right hand, bend forward and catch the big toe of the right foot with 2 first fingers of the right hand, turn the right hip back, left hip forward slightly engaging the legs. Raise the left arm pointing upwards, open the chest, keeping the shoulders broad and the neck long. Take 5 breaths with sound. Dhristi left middle finger

3. Trini inhale – bring your gaze back to the right toe and come back to upright, arms out-stretched turn feet back to parallel.

4. Chatwari exhale – turn left foot forward back foot 45 degrees, left heel should be in line with the middle of the arch of the right foot, looking into the middle finger of the left hand, bend and catch the big toe of the left foot with the 2 first fingers of the left hand, turn the left hip back right hip forward slightly engaging the legs. Raise the right arm pointing upwards, open the chest, keeping the shoulders broad and the neck Long. Take 5 breaths with sound. Dhristi right middle finger.

5. Pancha inhale – bring your gaze back to the left toe and come back to upright arms out-stretched, turn feet back to parallel.

Continue into next asana.

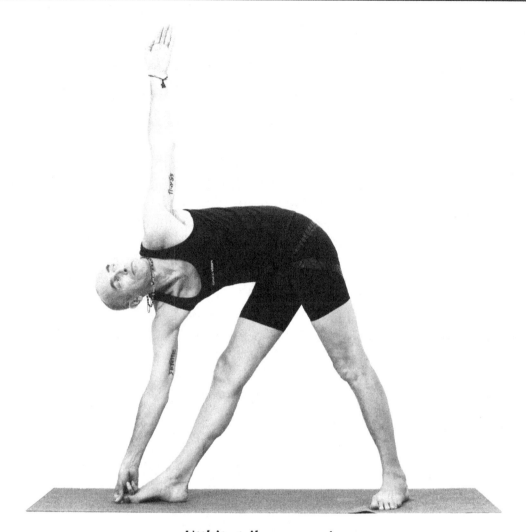

Utthita trikonasana A

MODIFICATION

If you can't catch your toes, catch your ankles or calves

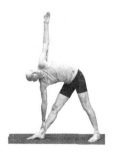

UTTHITA TRIKONASANA B – REVOLVED TRIANGLE POSE

1. Dwe exhale – turn right foot forward, back foot at 45 degrees, right heel should be in line with the middle of the arch of the left foot, bring the left hand over placing it to the right side of the right foot, raise the right hand upwards opening the chest keeping the shoulders broad and the neck long. Take 5 breaths with sound. Dhristi right middle finger

2. Trini inhale – bring your gaze back to the right toe and Come back to upright, arms outstretched, turn feet back to parallel.

3. Chatwari exhale – turn left foot forward back foot at 45 degrees, left heel should be in line with the middle of the arch of the right foot, bring the right hand over placing it to the left side of the left foot, raise the right hand upwards opening the chest keeping the shoulders broad and the neck long. Take 5 breaths with sound. Dhristi left middle finger.

4. Pancha inhale – bring your gaze back to the left toe and come back to upright, arms outstretched, turn feet back to parallel.

5. Exhale – jump or step back to front of the mat, lower the hands stand tall. Samasthiti

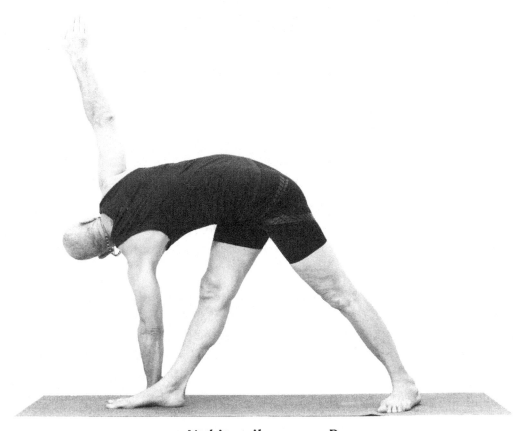

Utthita trikonasana B

MODIFICATION

If you can't catch your toes, catch your ankles or calves.

UTTHITA PARSVAKONASANA A – EXTENDED SIDE ANGLE POSE

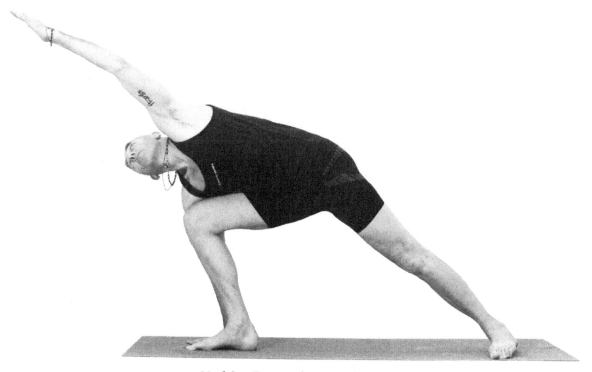

Utthita Parsvakonasana A

1. Ekam inhale - jump or step to the right hand-side, arms out stretched, feet should be approximately 4 feet apart, right foot pointing forward, back foot at 45 degrees. Right heel should be in line with the middle of the arch of the left foot

2. Dwe exhale - reach forward bending the knee to 90 degrees, lower the right hand to the floor on the outside of the right foot, bring the left hand over making a straight line from the left leg continuing up the left arm. Open the chest and torso, push down into the floor with the outside of the left foot. Make sure to keep the right thigh pointing straight forwards. Take 5 breaths with sound. Dhristi left middle finger.

3. Trini inhale - come back to upright arms out stretched, turn feet back to parallel.

4. Chatwari exhale - left foot pointing forward, back foot at 45 degrees. Left heel should be in line with the middle of the arch of the right foot. Reach forward bending the knee to 90 degrees. lower the left hand to the floor on the outside of the left foot, bring the right hand over making a straight line from the right leg continuing up the right arm. Push down into the floor with the outside of the right foot opening the chest and torso. Take 5 breaths with sound. Dhristi right finger.

5. Pancha inhale - come back to upright arms out stretched, turn feet back to parallel.

Continue into the next asana.

MODIFICATION

If you can't lower your hand to the floor let your elbow rest on your knee.

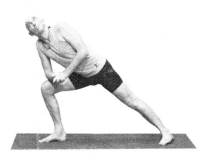

UTTHITA PARSVAKONASANA B – REVOLVED SIDE ANGLE POSE

1. Dwe exhale – turn to the right side, right foot pointing forward back foot at 45 degrees, right heel should be in line with the middle of the arch of the left foot, bend the right knee to 90 degrees, thigh pointing forward. Bring the left arm to the outside of the right knee, twisting the torso, hand to floor, raise the right arm making a straight line from the leg up the arm, open chest and torso. Take 5 breaths with sound. Dhristi right middle finger.

2. Trini inhale - come back to upright arms out stretched, turn feet back to parallel.

3. Chatwari exhale - turn to the left side, left foot pointing forward back foot 45 degrees, left heel should be in line with the middle of the arch of the right foot, bend the left knee to 90 degrees, thigh pointing forward. Bring the right arm to the outside of the left knee hand to floor, raise the left arm making a straight line from the leg up the arm, open chest and torso. Take 5 breaths with sound. Dhristi left middle finger

4. Pancha inhale - come back to upright arms out stretched, turn feet back to parallel.

5. Exhale - jump or step back to front of the mat, lower the hands, stand tall. Samasthiti.

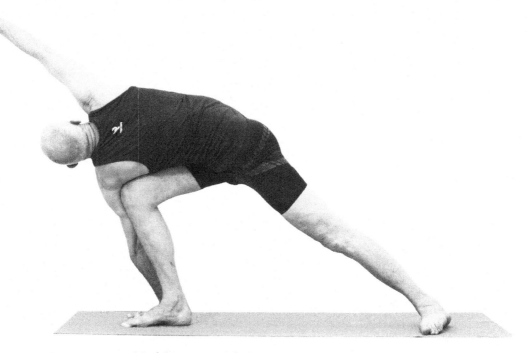

Utthita Parsvakonasana B

MODIFICATION

If you can't get your arm to the outside of your knee, let your shoulder rest on your knee bringing your hands into prayer position. Feel the twist and opening of the chest.

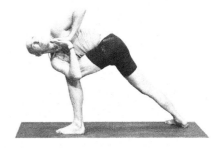

PRASARITA PADOTTANASANA A – WIDE LEG FORWARD BEND

1. Ekam inhale - jump or step to the right hand side, feet about 4ft apart, feet pointing straight forward or slightly inverted, hands on waist.

2. Dwe exhale – fold forward, drop the hands to the floor in line with your feet. Inhale – raise your head,

3. Trini exhale – fold forward finding space in your hips, straight legs, Take 5 breaths with sound. Dhristi tip of the nose.

4. Chatwari inhale – head up only, exhale there.

5. Pancha inhale - come back up, hands on waist. Exhale.

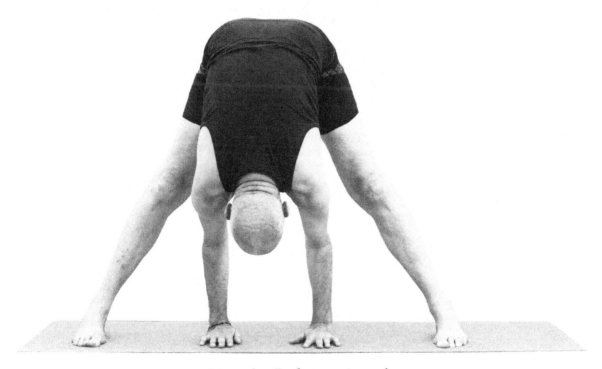

Prasarita Padottanasana A

PRASARITA PADOTTANASANA B

1. Ekam inhale - arms out stretched.

2. Dwe exhale - hands on waist, inhale there open chest.

3. Trini exhale - fold forward finding space in your hips, straight legs, keep hands on waist, Take 5 Breaths with sound. Dhristi tip of the nose.

4. Chatwari inhale - come back up, hands on waist, exhale there.

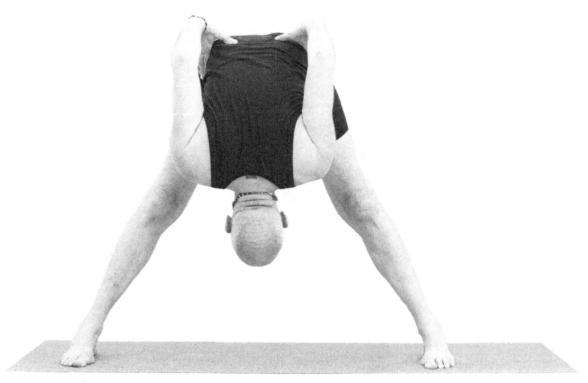

Prasarita Padottanasana B

PRASARITA PADOTTANASANA C

1. Ekam inhale– arms outstretched.

2. Dwe exhale – catch the hands behind the back, inhale open chest.

3. Trini exhale - bend forward. Take 5 breaths with sound. Dhristi tip of the nose.

4. Chatwari inhale - come back up hands on waist, exhale,

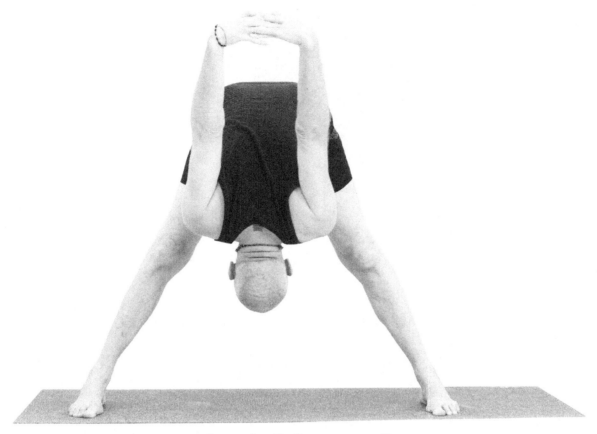

Prasarita Padottanasana C

PRASARITA PADOTTANASANA D

1. Ekam inhale - hands on waist

2. Dwe exhale – fold forward, catch the big toes with first two fingers. inhale raise the head

3. Trini exhale - fold forward, head to floor. Take 5 breaths with sound. Dhristi tip of the nose.

4. Chatwari inhale - head up only, open chest, exhale there.

5. Pancha inhale – come back up hands on waist.

6. exhale - jump or step back to the front of the mat Samasthiti.

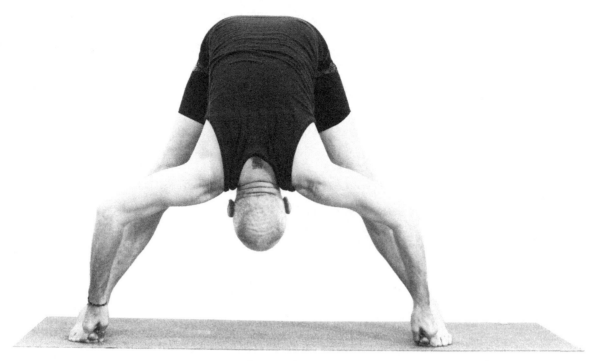

Prasarita Padottanasana D

MODIFICATION FOR A, B, C, D

If you can't lower your hands to the floor, put them on your thigh and fold forward, lowering your hands down the legs as far as you can.

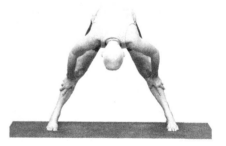

PARSVOTTANASANA – INTENSE SIDE STRETCH POSE

1. Ekam inhale – jump or step to the right hand side, feet 2ft apart, Right foot pointing forward, left foot at 45 degrees, bring the hands together behind the back in reverse prayer position, square hips, square shoulders.

2. Dwe exhale - fold forward, chin to knee. Take 5 breaths with sound. Dhristi right big toe.

3. Trini inhale – come back to upright, square hips, square shoulders.

4. Chatwari exhale - turn to the left hand side, left foot pointing forward, right foot at 45 degrees, fold forward, chin to knee. Take 5 breaths with sound. Dhristi left big toe.

5. Pancha inhale - come back to upright, square hips square shoulders.

6. Exhale – jump or step back to front of the mat release the hands. Samasthiti.

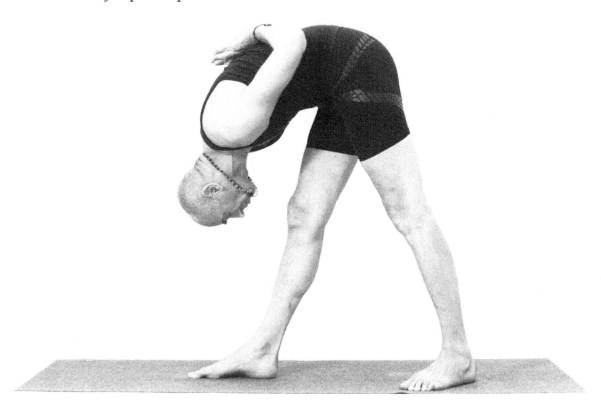

Parsvottanasana

MODIFICATION

If you can't bring your hands into reverse prayer, catch the elbows with hands.

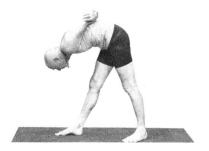

UTTHITA HASTA PADANGUSTHASANA – EXTENDED HAND TO TOE POSE

1. Ekam inhale – raise the right leg, catch the big toe with the first 2 fingers of the right hand, left hand on waist.

2. Dwe exhale – bend forward, touch chin to the knee. Take 5 breaths with sound. Dhristi right toe.

3. Trini inhale - come back to upright don't release the toe.

4. Chatwari exhale – bring the right leg out to the right hand side, opening the hip, extending the inner thigh, bandhas engaged, look over the left shoulder. Take 5 breaths with sound. Dhristi into the distance.

5. Pancha inhale - bring the right leg back to centre.

6. Shat exhale – bend forward, touch chin to knee.

7. Sapta inhale – come back to upright, release the toe, both hands on waist, point the toes, balance. Take 5 breaths with sound. Dhristi toe.

Exhale – lower the right leg to the ground.

8. Hastu inhale – raise the left leg catch the big toe with the first 2 fingers of the left hand, right hand on waist.

9. Nava exhale – bend forward, touch chin to the knee. Take 5 breaths with sound. Dhristi toe.

10. Dasa inhale - come back to upright don't release the toe.

11. Eka dasa exhale – bring the left leg out to the left hand side, opening the hip, extending the inner thigh, look over the right shoulder. Take 5 breaths with sound. Dhristi into the distance.

12. Dwe dasa Inhale - bring the left leg back to centre.

13. Trio dasa exhale – bend forward, touch chin to knee.

14. Chatur dasa inhale – come back to upright, release the toe, both hands on waist, point the toes, balance. Take 5 breaths with sound. Dhristi toes.

Exhale – lower the left leg to the ground, Samasthiti

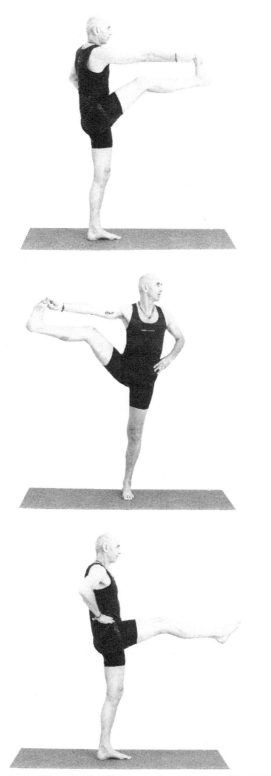

Utthita Hasta Padangusthasana A, B & C

MODIFICATION

Instead of catching your toe, raise your knee, hand on knee, take 5 breaths, exhale knee out to the right, hand on knee, look over left shoulder 5 breaths, inhale back to centre, extend the leg both hands on waist take 5 breaths.

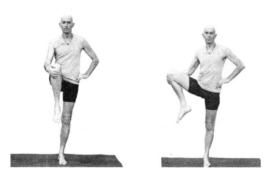

ARDHA BADHA PADMOTTANASANA – HALF BOUND LOTUS FORWARD FOLD POSE

1. Ekam inhale – take the right leg in to half lotus position, catch the right hand behind the back catching the right big toe.

2. Dwe exhale – fold forward, drop the left hand to the floor at the outside of the left foot. Take 5 breaths with sound. Dhristi left big toe.

3. Trini inhale – head up only, exhale there.

4. Chatwari inhale - come all the way up to standing

5. Pancha exhale – release the right leg.

6. Shat inhale – take the left leg in to half lotus position, catch the left hand behind the back catching the left big toe.

7. Sapta exhale – fold forward, drop the right hand to the floor at the outside of the right foot. Take 5 breaths with sound. Dhristi right big toe

8. Hastu inhale – head up only, exhale there.

9. Nava inhale - come all the way up to standing

10. Exhale – release the left leg, Samasthiti.

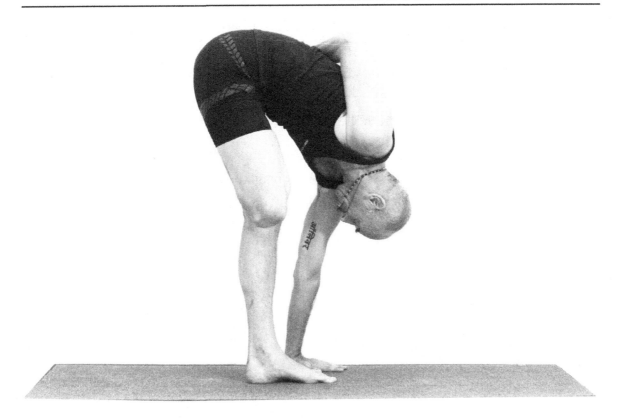

Ardha Badha Padmottanasana

MODIFICATION

If you do not have the confidence to 'catch' and go down with one hand, bring the right foot as high as possible into half lotus position, fold forward bringing both hands to the ground.

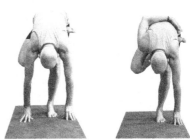

Once you are confident with this, you can start to bring one hand round the back and fold forward with one hand to the floor. A towel can be used to allow you to catch the foot, intensifying the stretch.

UTKATASANA – CHAIR POSE

1. Ekam inhale – raise the arms hands together, stretch tall lifting from the elbows extending the armpits and side trunk.

2. Dwe exhale – fold forward from the hips extending the hands to the floor.

3. Trini inhale – head up only.

4. Chatwari exhale – jump back to chaturanga, plank position.

5. Pancha inhale – raise the chest look up, upward facing dog.

6. Shat exhale - raise the hips, downward facing dog.

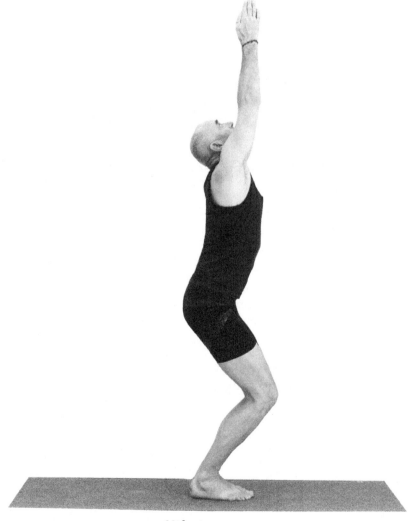

Utkatasana

7. Sapta inhale – jump forward, bend the knees, raise both arms, turn in the triceps, lift from the elbows, hands together. Hands, shoulders, hips, ankles in a straight line. Take 5 breaths with sound. Dhristi thumbs.

8. Hastu inhale - straighten legs.

9. Nava exhale – fold forward hands to floor, jump back to chaturanga, plank position.

10. Dasa inhale – raise the chest look up, upward facing dog.

11. Eka dasa exhale – raise the hips, downward facing dog.

Continue into next asana

VIRABHADRASANA A – WARRIOR POSE

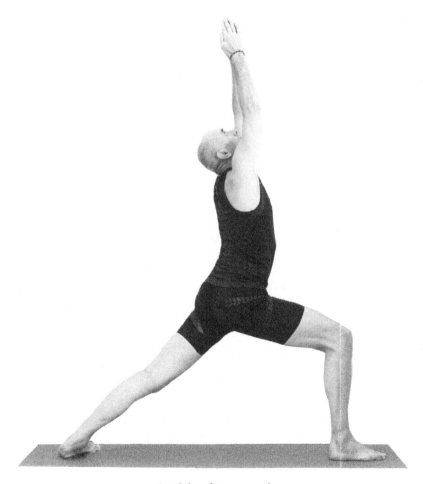

Virabhadrasana A

1. Sapta inhale – bring right foot forward, turn left foot in to 45*. Bend the right knee, bringing the knee over the foot. Raise the hands above the head lifting from the elbows to give maximum stretch, chest square. Take 5 breaths with sound. Dhristi thumbs

2. Inhale - straighten the right leg, turn to left hand side, left foot pointing forward, right foot at 45 degrees.

3. Hastu exhale - bend the left knee, bringing the knee over the foot, Raise the hands above the head lifting from the elbows to give maximum stretch, chest square. Take 5 breaths with sound. Dhristi thumbs.

4. Inhale.

Continue into next asana

MODIFICATION

Don't bend your knee too far, stay within your comfort zone.

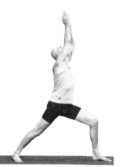

VIRABHADRASANA B

1. Nava exhale - open the arms parallel to the floor in line with the legs, open chest Take 5 breaths with sound. Dhristi middle finger left hand

2. Inhale - straighten the left leg, turn to right hand side, right foot pointing forward left foot 45* keep the arms outstretched.

3. Dasa exhale - bend the right knee, bringing the knee over the foot, arms outstretched, chest open. Take 5 breaths with sound. Dhristi middle finger right hand.

4. Eka dasa inhale – take both hands to the floor on each side of the right foot,

5. Dwe dasa chatwari exhale - jump back to chaturanga, plank position.

6. Trio dasa inhale – raise the chest look up, (upward facing dog).

7. Chatur dasa exhale - raise the hips, (downward facing dog).

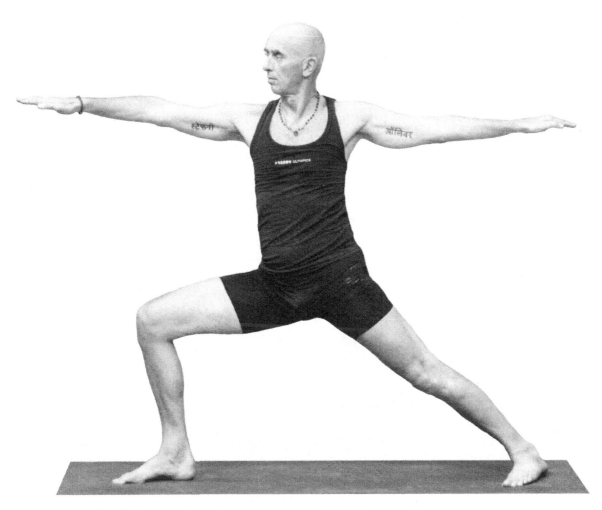

Virabhadrasana B

MODIFICATION

Don't bend the knee too far, stay within your comfort zone.

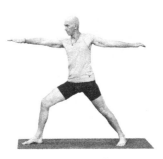

SITTING SERIES OF ASANAS

DANDASANA – STAFF POSE

1. Sapta inhale – jump through to sitting position, straight legs, straight back. Place the hands at the side of the waist pressing down with the palms, shoulders open. Push forward with the heels, strong legs. Lower the chin, engage Jalandhara bandha, all 3 bandhas engaged. Take 5 breaths with sound. Dhristi nose.

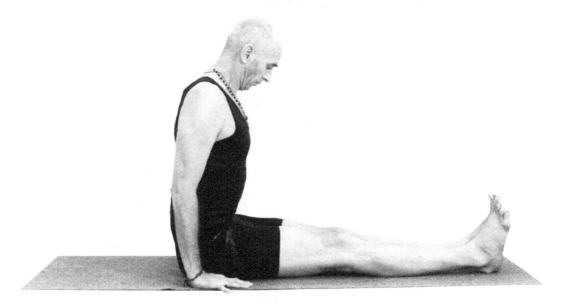

Dandasana

PACHIMATANASANA A - SEATED FORWARD BEND

1. Hastu inhale – catch the big toes with the first 2 fingers. Lengthen the spine, open the chest, head up.

2. Nava exhale – fold forward over uddiyana bandha chin to knee, maintaining length in the spine, open the elbows to the side opening the chest and shoulders. Take 5 breaths with sound. Dhristi toes

3. Dasa inhale – head up only, exhale there.

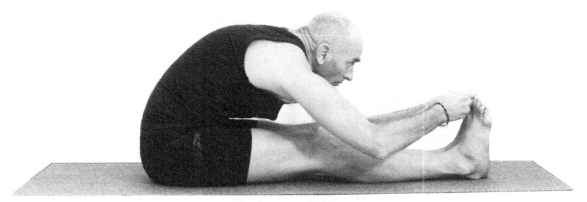

Pachimatanasana A

MODIFICATION

Catch your calf or ankles, bend from the hips over udiyana bandha, extend the chest.

PACHIMATANASANA B

1. Hastu inhale – catch the heels or bind catching the wrist with the hand, straight legs.

2. Nava exhale - fold forward over uddiyana bandha, chin to knee, maintaining length in the spine, open the elbows to the side, opening the chest and shoulders. Take 5 breaths with sound. Dhristi toes.

3. Dasa inhale – head up only, exhale there.

4. Eka dasa inhale - lift up

5. Dwe dasa chatwari exhale - jump back to chaturanga, plank position.

6. Trio dasa inhale - lift the chest (upward facing dog).

7. Chatur dasa exhale - raise the hips, (downward facing dog).

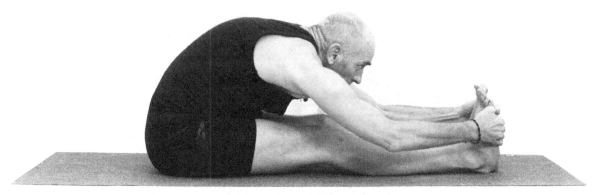

Pachimatanasana B

Modification: catch your calf or ankles, bend from your hips over udiyana bandha, extend your chest, open the elbows.

PURVATTANASANA – UPWARD FACING PLANK POSE

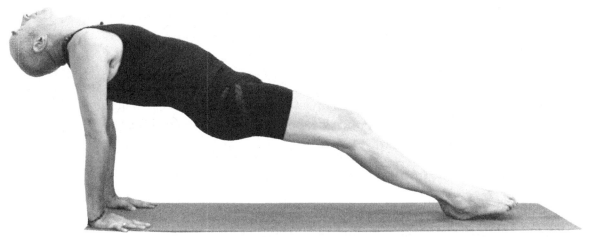

Purvattanasana

1. Sapta inhale - jump through to sitting straight legs. Exhale – Place the hands one foot back behind the hips, fingers facing forward

2. Hastu inhale – raise the hips, push the feet flat to the floor, roll the thighs in, relax the neck. Try to keep the full body in a straight line. Take 5 breaths with sound. Dhristi nose.

3. Nava Exhale - lower the body down.

4. Dasa inhale – lift up

5. Eka dasa chatwari exhale - jump back to chaturanga, plank position.

6. Dwe dasa inhale - lift the chest (upward facing dog).

7. Trio dasa exhale - raise the hips (downward facing dog).

MODIFICATION

Bring the feet closer and bend the knees to 90 degrees, inhale up, heels together.

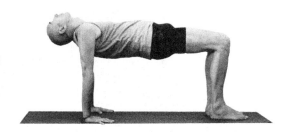

ARDHA BADHA PADMA PACHIMATANASANA – HALF BOUND LOTUS FORWARD BEND

1. Sapta inhale – jump through to sitting take the right leg into half lotus position, bind the right arm round the back and catch the right foot, square shoulders, maintain length in the torso.

2. Hastu exhale – fold forward leading with the chest, chin to knee, straight spine, catch left foot with the left hand, do not rest the arm on the floor. 5 breaths with sound. Dhristi left big toe.

3. Nava inhale – head up only, exhale there.

4. Dasa inhale - lift up

5. Eka dasa chatwari exhale - jump back to chaturanga, plank position.

6. Dwe dasa inhale - lift the chest (upward facing dog).

7. Trio dasa exhale - raise the hips, (downward facing dog).

8. Chatur dasa inhale - jump through to sitting, take the left leg into half lotus position, bind the left arm round the back and catch the left foot, square shoulders, maintain length in the torso.

9. Pancha dasa exhale - fold forward Take 5 breaths with sound. Dhristi right big toe.

10. Sho dasa inhale - head up only, exhale there.

11. Sapta dasa inhale - lift up.

12. Hastu dasa chatwari exhale - jump back to chaturanga, plank position

13. Ekona vimshatih inhale - lift the chest (upward facing dog).

14. Vimshatih exhale - raise the hips (downward facing dog).

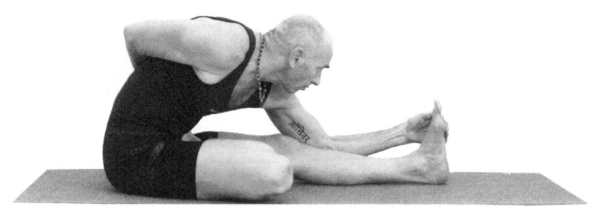

Ardha Baddha Padma Paschimottanasana

MODIFICATIONS

Bring your right leg in to half lotus, fold forward with both hands to try catch the foot.

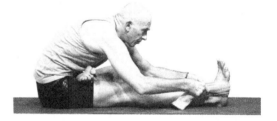

If you can't catch your right foot with your right hand use a towel to help catch, fold forward.

TIRYANGMUKHA EKAPADA PACHIMATANASANA – THREE LIMBED FORWARD POSE

1. Sapta inhale - jump through to sitting, take the right leg back, foot pointing backwards, square shoulders maintain length in the torso.

2. Hastu exhale – fold forward chin to knee, leading with the chest, straight spine, catch the left foot with both hands or bind catching the wrist with the hand, resist the urge to lean over to the left side leading with the left shoulder, Open the elbows to allow a deeper fold, do not rest the arms on the floor. Take 5 breaths with sound. Dhristi left big toe.

3. Nava inhale – head up only, exhale there.

4. Dasa inhale - lift up

5. Eka dasa chatwari exhale - jump back to chaturanga, plank position.

6. Dwe dasa inhale - lift the chest (upward facing dog).

7. Trio dasa exhale - raise the hips, (downward facing dog).

8. Chatur dasa inhale - jump through to sitting, take the left leg back, square shoulders maintain length in the torso.

9. Pancha dasa exhale - fold forward chin to knee, leading with the chest, straight spine, catch the right foot with both hands or bind. Take 5 breaths with sound. Dhristi left big toe.

10. Sho dasa inhale - head up only, exhale there.

11. Sapta dasa inhale - lift up.

12. Hastu dasa chatwari exhale - jump back to chaturanga, plank position.

13. Ekona vimshatih inhale - lift the chest, (upward facing dog).

14. Vimshatih exhale - raise the hips, (downward facing dog).

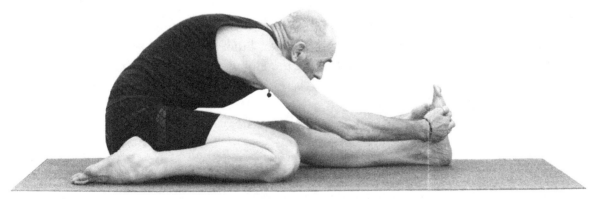

Tiryangmukha Ekapada Pachimatanasana

MODIFICATIONS

Fold your towel and place it under the sitting bone of the straight leg.

If you can't catch your feet, catch your ankle or calf.

JANUSIRSASANA A – HEAD TO KNEE POSE

1. Sapta inhale - jump through to sitting, bring the right heel to the inside of the left leg, heel towards the anus, knee open out to the right side, square hips, square shoulders maintain length in the torso.

2. Hastu exhale – fold forward chin to knee, leading with the chest, straight spine, catch the left foot with both hands or bind catching the wrist with the hand, as you fold forward the right heel should put pressure on the anus. Open the elbows to allow a deeper fold, do not rest the arms on the floor. Take 5 breaths with sound. Dhristi left big toe.

3. Nava inhale – head up only, exhale there.

4. Dasa inhale - lift up.

5. Eka dasa chatwari exhale - jump back to chaturanga, plank position.

6. Dwe dasa inhale - lift the chest, (upward facing dog).

7. Trio dasa exhale - raise the hips, (downward facing dog).

8. Chatur dasa inhale - jump through to sitting, bring the left heel to the inside of the right leg, heel towards the anus, knee open out to the right side, square hips, square shoulders.

9. Pancha dasa exhale – fold forward chin to knee, leading with the chest, straight spine, catch the right foot with the both hands or bind, as you fold forward the right heel should put pressure on the anus. Open the elbows to allow a deeper fold. Take 5 breaths with sound. Dhristi right big toe.

10. Sho dasa inhale - head up only, exhale there.

11. Sapta dasa inhale - lift up.

12. Hastu dasa chatwari exhale - jump back to chaturanga, plank position.

13. Ekona vimshatih inhale - lift the chest, (upward facing dog).

14. Vimshatih exhale - raise the hips, (downward facing dog).

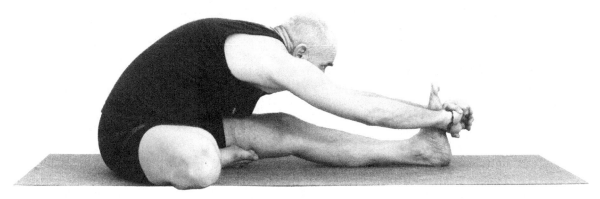

Janusirsasana A

MODIFICATION

If you can't catch the feet, catch your ankles or calf muscles or use a towel to intensify the stretch.

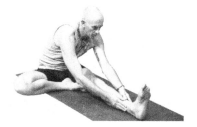

JANUSIRSASANA B

1. Sapta inhale - jump through to sitting, bring the right foot up as in A, but this time the heel goes behind the anus, foot pointing forward, knee open out to the right side, square hips, square shoulders maintain length in the torso.

2. Hastu exhale – fold forward chin to knee, leading with the chest, straight spine, catch the left foot with the hands or bind catching the wrist with the hand, open the elbows to allow a deeper fold, do not rest the arms on the floor. Take 5 breaths with sound. Dhristi left toe.

3. Nava inhale – head up only, exhale there.

4. Dasa inhale – lift up.

5. Eka dasa chatwari exhale – jump back to chaturanga, plank position.

6. Dwe dasa inhale – lift the chest, (upward facing dog).

7. Trio dasa exhale – raise the hips, (downward facing dog).

8. Chatur dasa inhale - jump through, bring the left heel behind the anus, foot pointing forward, knee open out to the right side, square hips.

9. Pancha dasa exhale – fold forward leading with the chest, straight spine, catch the right foot with both hands or bind, chin to knee. Take 5 breaths with sound. Dhristi toe.

10. Sho dasa inhale – head up only, exhale there.

11. Sapta dasa inhale - lift up.

12. Hastu dasa chatwari exhale - jump back to chaturanga, plank position.

13. Ekona vimshatih inhale - lift the chest, (upward facing dog).

14. Vimshatih exhale - raise the hips, (downward facing dog).

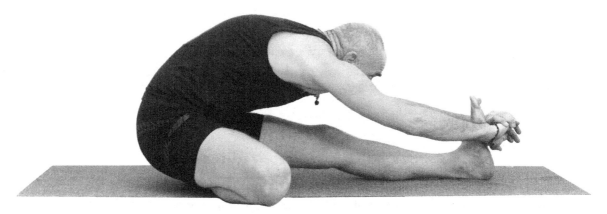

Janusirsasana B

MODIFICATION

If you can't catch the feet, catch your ankles or calf muscles or use a towel to intensify the stretch.

JANUSIRSASANA C

1. Sapta inhale - jump through to sitting, bring the right heel onto the left thigh, twist the ankle, toes to the floor, knee open out to the right side, square hips, square shoulders maintain length in the torso.

2. Hastu exhale – fold forward chin to knee, leading with the chest, straight spine, catch the left foot with the both hands or bind catching the wrist with the hand, open the elbows to allow a deeper fold, do not rest the arms on the floor. Take 5 breaths with sound. Dhristi left toe.

3. Nava Inhale – head up only, exhale there.

4. Dasa inhale – lift up.

5. Eka dasa chatwari exhale – jump back to chaturanga, plank position.

6. Dwe dasa inhale – lift the chest, (upward facing dog).

7. Trio dasa exhale – raise the hips, (downward facing dog).

8. Chatur dasa inhale – jump through to sitting, bring the left heel onto the right thigh, twist the ankle, toes to the floor, knee open out to the left side, square hips, square shoulders maintain length in the torso.

9. Pancha dasa exhale – fold forward leading with the chest, straight spine, catch the right foot with the both hands or bind, Open the elbows to allow a deeper fold. Take 5 breaths with sound. Dhristi right toe.

10. Sho dasa inhale – head up only, exhale there.

11. Sapta dasa - lift up.

12. Hastu dasa chatwari exhale - jump back to chaturanga, plank position.

13. Ekona vimshatih inhale - lift the chest, (upward facing dog).

14. Vimshatih exhale - raise the hips, (downward facing dog).

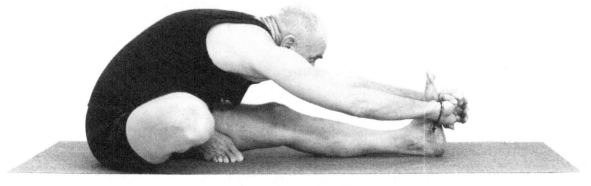

Janusirsasana C

MODIFICATION

First get used to the ankle and toes bending into position, don't fold forward, feel the stretch in the foot, take 5 breaths there. Slowly increase flexibility by bending forward a little more each day.

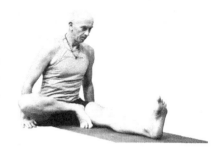

MARICHASANA A – POSE DEDICATED TO SAGE MARICHI

1. Sapta inhale - jump through to sitting, raise the right knee, leave space between the foot and the thigh. Raise the right arm lengthening the torso, stretch forward taking the right arm round the right leg, bring the left arm round the back catching the right hand.

2. Hastu exhale - fold forward chin to knee, leading with the chest, straight spine. Take 5 breaths with sound. Dhristi big toe of left foot.

3. Nava inhale – head up only, exhale there.

4. Dasa inhale - lift up.

5. Eka dasa chatwari exhale - jump back to chaturanga, plank position.

6. Dwe dasa inhale - lift the chest, (upward facing dog).

7. Trio dasa exhale - raise the hips, (downward facing dog).

8. Chatur dasa inhale - jump through to sitting, raise the left knee, leave space between the foot and the thigh. Raise the left arm lengthening the torso, stretch forward taking the left arm round the left leg, bring the right arm round the back catching the left hand.

9. Pancha dasa exhale - fold forward leading with the chest, straight spine, chin to knee. Take 5 breaths with sound. Dhristi big toe of right foot.

10. Sho dasa Inhale – head up only, exhale there.

11. Sapta dasa inhale - lift up.

12. Hastu dasa chatwari exhale – jump back to chaturanga, plank position.

13. Ekona vimshatih inhale -lift the chest, (upward facing dog).

14. Vimshatih exhale - raise the hips, (downward facing dog).

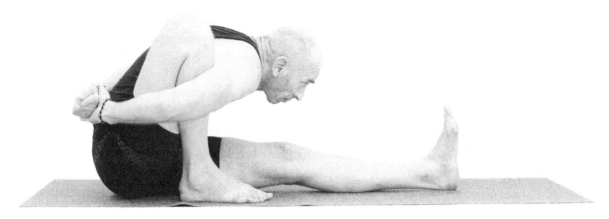

Marichasana A

MODIFICATION

If you can't catch the hands together, use a towel.

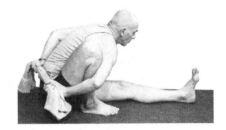

MARICHASANA B

1. Sapta inhale - jump through to sitting, bring the left leg into half lotus, raise the right knee, raise the right arm lengthening the torso, stretch forward taking the right arm round the right leg, bring the left arm round the back catching the right hand.

2. Hastu exhale - fold forward, chin to the floor. Take 5 breaths with sound. Dhristi tip of the nose.

3. Nava Inhale – head up only, exhale there.

4. Dasa inhale - lift up.

5. Eka dasa chatwari exhale - jump back to chaturanga, plank position.

6. Dwe dasa inhale - lift the chest, (upward facing dog).

7. Trio dasa exhale - raise the hips, (downward facing dog).

8. Chatur dasa inhale - jump through to sitting, bring the right leg into half lotus, raise the left knee, raise the left arm lengthening the torso, stretch forward taking the left arm round the left leg. Bring the right arm round the back catching the left hand.

9. Pancha dasa exhale - fold forward, chin to the floor. Take 5 breaths with sound. Dhristi tip of the nose.

10. Sho dasa inhale – head up only, exhale there.

11. Sapta dasa inhale - lift up.

12. Hastu dasa chatwari exhale - jump back to chaturanga, plank position.

13. Ekona vimshatih inhale - lift the chest, (upward facing dog).

14. Vimshatih exhale - raise the hips, (downward facing dog).

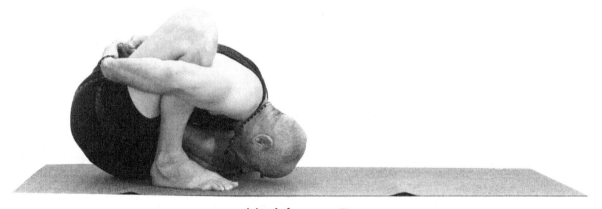

Marichasana B

MODIFICATIONS

Bring the left leg into half lotus raise the right knee, catch the knee with both hands, take 5 breaths.

If you have trouble with half lotus bring left leg under the right knee, fold forward, take 5 breaths.

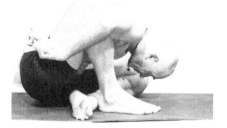

MARICHASANA C

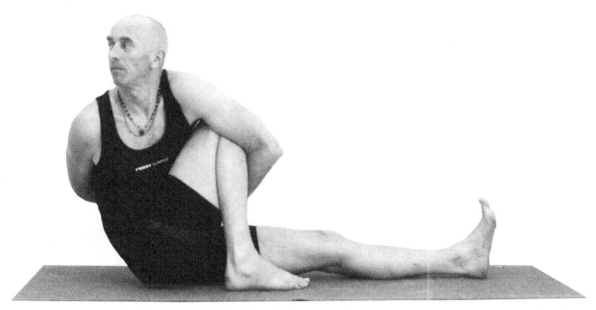

Marichasana C

1. Sapta inhale - jump through to sitting, raise the right knee, leave space between the foot and the thigh. Raise the left hand lengthening the torso, twist from the waist, take the left arm round the outside of the right leg, bend the elbow taking the arm back, bring the right arm round the back catching the left hand. Open the chest and shoulders lengthening the side trunk, look over the right shoulder. Take 5 breaths with sound. Dhristi into the distance

2. Hastu inhale – lift up.

3. Nava chatwari exhale - jump back to chaturanga, plank position.

4. Dasa inhale - lift the chest, (upward facing dog).

5. Eka dasa exhale - raise the hips, (downward facing dog).

6. Dwe dasa inhale - jump through to sitting, raise the left knee, leave space between the foot and the thigh. Raise the right hand lengthening the torso, twist from the waist, take the right arm round the outside of the left leg, bend the elbow taking the arm back, bring the left arm round the back catching the left hand. Open the chest and shoulders lengthening the side trunk, look over the left shoulder. Take 5 breaths with sound. Dhristi into the distance

7. Trio dasa Inhale - lift up

8. Chatur dasa chatwari exhale - jump back to chaturanga, plank position

9. Pancha dasa inhale - lift the chest, (upward facing dog).

10. Sho dasa exhale - raise the hips, (downward facing dog).

MODIFICATIONS

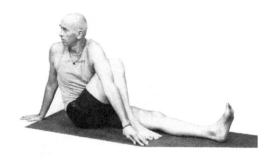

It is quite difficult to combine the jump through and the bind on one single breath, so take an extra breath after jumping through.

If you have trouble bending the elbow and catching, leave the right hand on the floor, with left arm outside the right knee.

MARICHASANA D

1. Sapta inhale - jump through to sitting, take the left leg in to half lotus position, raise the right knee, raise the left hand lengthening the torso, twist from the waist, take the left arm round the outside of the right leg, bend the elbow taking the arm back, bring the right arm round the back catching the left hand. Open the chest and shoulders lengthening the side trunk, look over the right shoulder. Take 5 breaths with sound. Dhristi into the distance.

2. Hastu inhale - lift up.

3. Nava chatwari exhale - jump back to chaturanga, plank position.

4. Dasa inhale - lift the chest, (upward facing dog).

5. Eka dasa exhale - raise the hips, (downward facing dog).

6. Dwe dasa inhale - jump through to sitting, take right leg into half lotus position, raise the left knee, raise the right hand lengthening the torso, twist from the waist, take the right arm round the outside of the left leg, bend the elbow taking the arm back, bring the left arm round the back catching the left hand. Open the chest and shoulders lengthening the side trunk, look over the left shoulder. Take 5 breaths with sound. Dhristi into the distance.

7. Trio dasa inhale - lift up.

8. Chatur dasa chatwari exhale - jump back to chaturanga, plank position.

9. Pancha dasa inhale - lift the chest, (upward facing dog).

10. Sho dasa exhale - raise the hips, (downward facing dog).

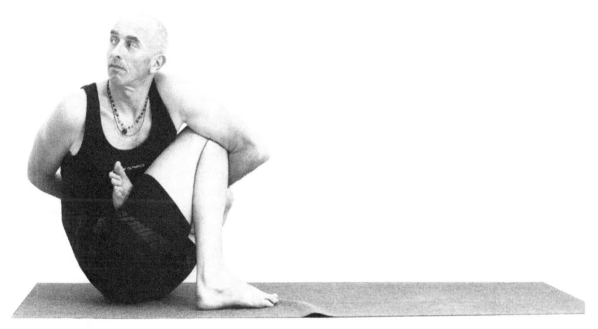

Marichasana D

MODIFICATIONS

Bring the left leg into half lotus, raise the right knee, take the right arm back, with left arm outside the right knee, take 5 breaths.

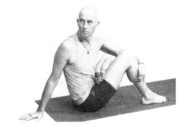

If you have trouble with half lotus, bring left leg under the right knee, try to catch the hands, take 5 breaths.

NAVASANA – BOAT POSE

1. Sapta inhale - jump through, raise the legs feet pointing forward just above eye level, arms straight and parallel to the floor, palms facing each other, lift the chest. Take 5 breaths with sound. Dhristi, tip of the big toe. Exhale down.

2. Hastu inhale - lift the buttocks from the floor with crossed legs, exhale down.

3. Sapta inhale - again up to navasana position 5 breaths, repeat 4 more times.

4. Nava chatwari exhale - jump back to chaturanga, plank position.

5. Dasa inhale - lift the chest, (upward facing dog).

6. Eka dasa exhale -raise the hips, (downward facing dog).

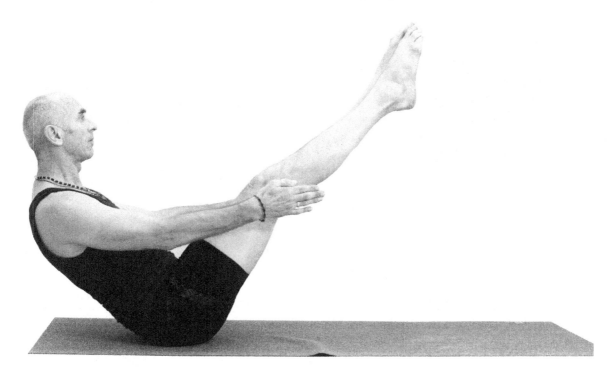

Navasana

MODIFICATION

If you are feeling too much strain with straight legs, bend the knees slightly, while keeping the arms outstretched,

If you get too tired catch the hands on legs.

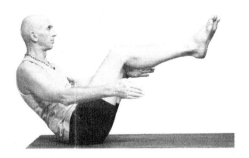

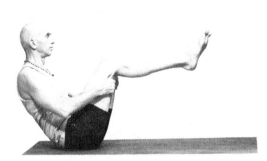

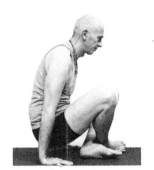

BHUJAPIDASANA – SHOULDER PRESSING POSE

1. Sapta inhale - jump the legs onto the upper arms, bend the legs and cross the ankles

2. Hastu exhale - lower the forehead to the floor, feet should not touch the floor. Take 5 breaths with sound. Dhristi tip of the nose

3. Nava inhale - raise the head and torso, exhale there.

4. Dasa inhale - release the legs, bring them into bakasana position.

5. Eka dasa chatwari exhale - jump back to chaturanga, plank position.

6. Dwe dasa inhale - lift the chest, (upward facing dog).

7. Trio dasa exhale - raise the hips, (downward facing dog).

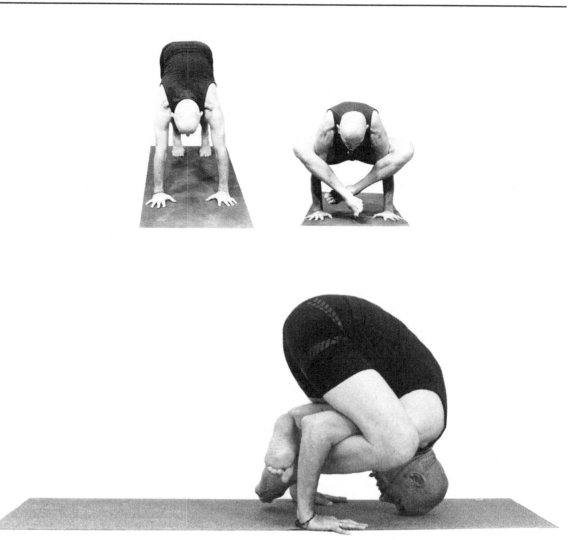

Bhujapidasana

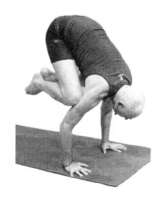

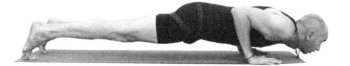

MODIFICATIONS

Sapta inhale - jump the feet to the outside of the hands then cross the legs, keeping the feet on the floor, lower down if possible, head to floor, take 5 breaths.

Dasa inhale - If you can't bring the legs back into bakasana walk the feet back and jump back vinyasa in your usual way.

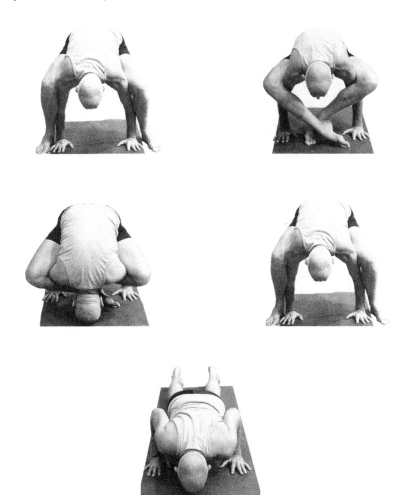

KURMASANA – TORTOISE POSE

1. Sapta inhale - jump the legs onto the upper arms with feet pointed, exhale - lower down to the floor, reach the arms out under the knees, chest forward, straighten the legs. Take 5 breaths with sound. Dhristi, tip of the nose.

Continue into the next asana.

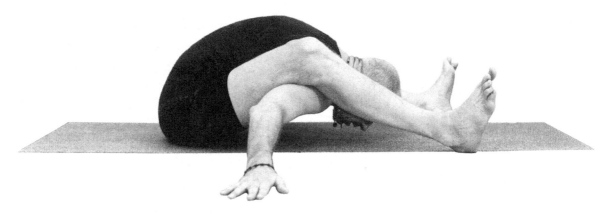

Kurmasana

MODIFICATION

Jump the feet to the outside of the hands, exhale lower down.

SUPTA KURMASANA – SLEEPING TORTOISE POSE.

1. Hastu exhale – catch the hands behind the back and lock the hands.

2. Nava inhale - cross the legs over the back of the neck or cross the ankles in front of the head. Take 5 breaths with sound. Dhristi tip of the nose.

3. Dasa inhale – release the hands to the floor, lift the torso and legs, exhale there.

4. Eka dasa inhale - bring the legs back to bakasana position.

5. Dwe dasa chatwari exhale - jump back to chaturanga, plank position.

6. Trio dasa inhale - lift the chest, (upward facing dog).

7. Chatur dasa exhale - raise the hips, (downward facing dog).

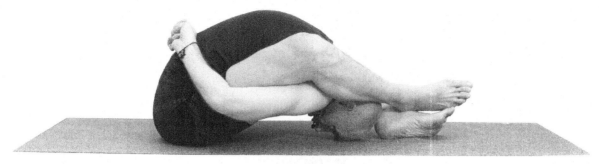

Supta Kurmasana

MODIFICATIONS

If you can't catch the hands together behind the back use a towel

If you can't cross the ankles you can bring the feet together as close as possible.

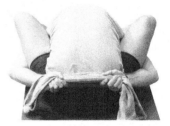

If you can't bring the legs back into bakasana, lift the torso and legs, exhale there. Then walk the feet back and jump back vinyasa in your usual way

GARBHA PINDASANA – WOMB EMBRYO POSE

1. Sapta inhale - jump through to sitting position, exhale there.

2. Hastu inhale – take the legs into Padmasana position, thread the arms through the legs in front of the feet, rest your chin in your hands. Take 5 breaths with sound. Dhristi nose.

3. Nava exhale - roll back, inhale come back up, each time make a small rotation, repeat 5 times making one full rotation. On the last roll inhale up, drop the hands to the floor.

Continue into the next asana.

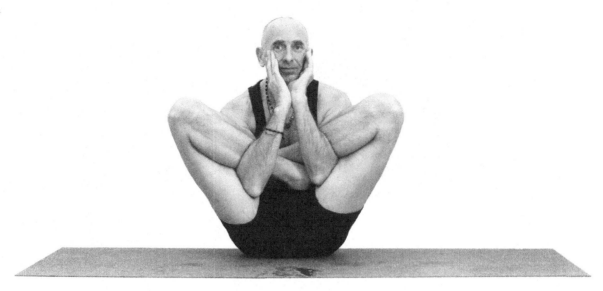

Garbha Pindasana

MODIFICATION

If you can't get your hands through, raise the knees and catch the hands round the knees. Take 5 breaths, then roll back.

If you can't do full lotus, cross your legs.

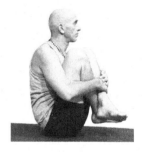

KUKKUTASANA – COCKEREL POSE

1. Nava inhale - lift, balancing on the hands. Take 5 breaths with sound. Dhristi nose. Exhale down release the arms.

2. Dasa inhale - lift up.

3. Eka dasa chatwari exhale - jump back to chaturanga, plank position.

4. Dwe dasa inhale - lift the chest, (upward facing dog).

5. Trio dasa exhale - raise the hips, (downward facing dog).

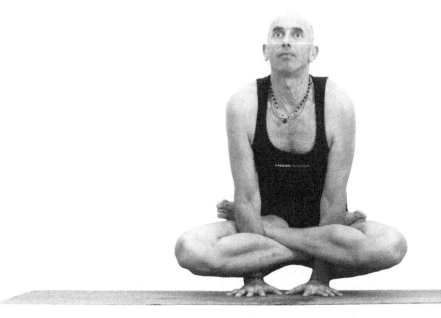

Kukkutasana

MODIFICATION:

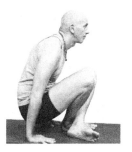

If you can't get your hands through, catch as in garbha pindasana modification and lift into Utplutih.

BADDHA KONASANA A – BOUND ANGLE POSE

1. Sapta inhale - jump through to sitting position, bring the feet together up towards groin, knees out to side, spread the balls of the feet with the thumbs, chest tall and open.

2. Hastu exhale - bend forward, straight back, chin to floor. Take 5 breaths with sound. Dhristi tip of the nose.

3. Nava inhale - come back to upright.

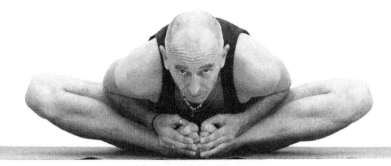

Baddha konasana A

BADDHA KONASANA B

1. Dasa exhale - touch the head to the toes, keep the balls of the feet open with the thumbs. Take 5 breaths with sound. Dhristi tip of the nose.

2. Eka dasa inhale - come back to upright, exhale.

3. Dwe dasa inhale - lift up.

4. Trio dasa chatwari exhale - jump back to chaturanga, plank position.

5. Chatur dasa inhale - lift the chest, (upward facing dog).

6. Pancha dasa exhale - raise the hips, (downward facing dog).

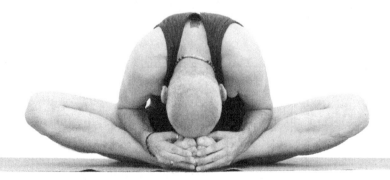

Baddha konasana B

MODIFICATION

Only bend forward to your own limit in both variations.

UPAVISTHA KONASANA A – WIDE ANGLE SEATED FORWARD BEND

1. Sapta inhale - jump through to sitting, spread the legs, catch outside of the feet with the hands, head up.

2. Hastu exhale - fold forward chin to floor. Take 5 breaths with sound. Dhristi tip of the nose.

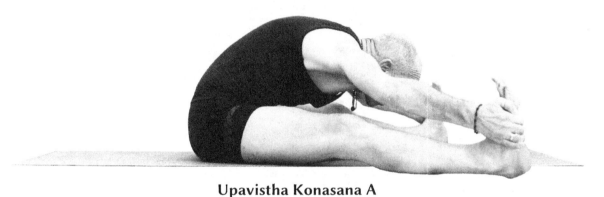

Upavistha Konasana A

Continue into Upavistha konasana B

MODIFICATIONS

If you can't catch the feet, hold the calf or ankles and bend forward.

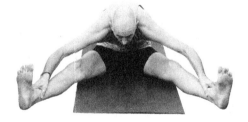

UPAVISTHA KONASANA B

3. Nava inhale - head up only, exhale there.

4. Dasa inhale up - raise straight legs, don't release the hands, point the feet extending from the inner thighs, look up. Take 5 breaths with sound. Dhristi up to space.

5. Eka dasa inhale - lift up.

6. Dwe dasa chatwari exhale - jump back to chaturanga, plank position.

7. Trio dasa inhale - lift the chest, (upward facing dog).

8. Chatur dasa exhale - raise the hips, (downward facing dog).

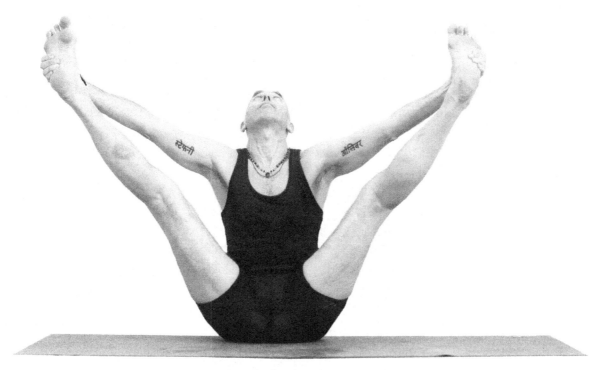

Upavistha Konasana B

MODIFICATION

If you can't catch the feet, catch the calf or ankles.

SUPTA KONASANA – RECLINING ANGLE POSE

1. Sapta inhale - jump through to sitting, lie down, exhale

2. Hastu inhale - take the legs back over the head, catch the big toes spread the legs. Take 5 breaths with sound. Dhristi nose.

3. Nava inhale - roll to upright exhale down don't stop, don't release the feet.

4. Dasa inhale - head up only, exhale there.

5. Eka dasa inhale - lift up.

6. Dwe dasa chatwari exhale - jump back to chaturanga plank position.

7. Trio dasa inhale - lift the chest, (upward facing dog).

8. Chatur dasa exhale – raise the hips, (downward facing dog).

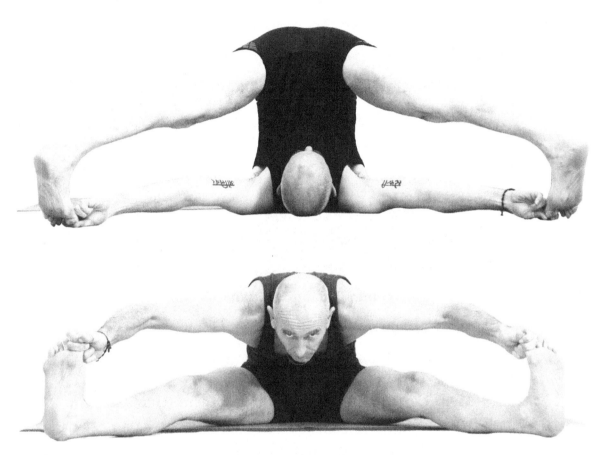

Supta Konasana

MODIFICATION

If you can't catch the feet, catch the calf or ankles.

SUPTA PADANGUSTHASANA – RECLINING BIG TOE POSE

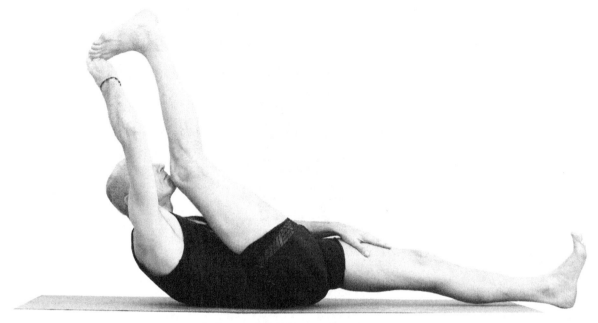

Supta Padangusthasana

1. Sapta inhale - jump through to sitting lie down, exhale.

2. Hastu inhale - raise the right leg catch the big toe with the right hand, straight legs, left hand on thigh.

3. Nava exhale - chin to knee, Take 5 breaths with sound. Dhristi nose

4. Dasa inhale - head down, don't release the toe.

5. Eka dasa exhale - take right leg out to the right side, straight leg, don't raise left hip from the floor, look over the left shoulder, use the weight of the right leg to open the hip and increase the stretch. Take 5 breaths with sound. Dhristi into distance over left shoulder.

6. Dwe dasa inhale - bring leg back to centre, straight leg.

7. Trio dasa exhale- chin to knee.

8. Chatur dasa inhale - head down.

9. Pancha dasa exhale - release the foot.

10. Sho dasa inhale - raise the left leg catch the big toe, right hand on thigh.

11. Sapta dasa exhale - chin to knee, Take 5 breaths with sound. Dhristi nose

12. Hastu dasa inhale - head down, don't release the toe,

13. Ekona vimshatih exhale - take left leg out to the left side, straight leg, look over the right shoulder, use the weight of the left leg to open the hip and increase the stretch. Take 5 breaths with sound. Dhristi into distance over right shoulder.

14. Vimshatih inhale - bring leg back to centre, straight leg.

15. Eka vimshatih exhale - chin to knee.

16. Dwe vimshatih inhale - head down.

17. Trio vimshatih exhale - release the foot.

18. Chatur vimshatih inhale, chakrasana, - Backward roll into chaturanga, plank position, exhale.

19. Pancha vimshatih inhale - lift the chest, (upward facing dog).

20. Shat vimshatih exhale - raise the hips, (downward facing dog).

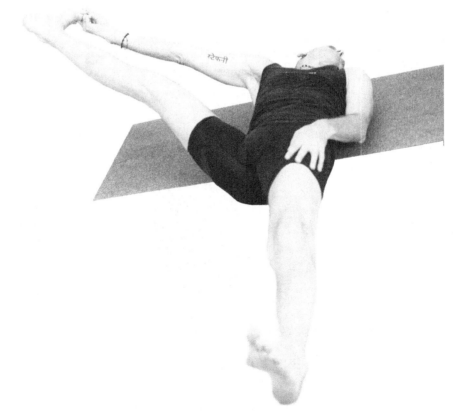

Supta Padangusthasana

MODIFICATION

If you can't catch with straight leg bend the knee slightly or use a towel to help intensify the stretch.

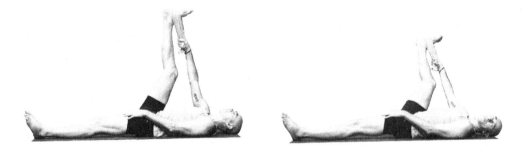

UBHAYA PADANGUSTHASANA – TWO FOOT POSE

1. Sapta inhale - jump through to sitting lie down, exhale.

2. Hastu Inhale - take the legs back over the head, catch the big toes, exhale there.

3. Nava Inhale – roll up into position, straight legs, point toes look up. Take 5 breaths with sound. Dhristi up to space.

4. Dasa inhale up.

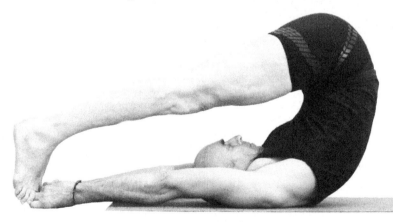

Ubhaya Padangusthasana

5. Eka dasa chatwari exhale - jump back to chaturanga, plank position.

6. Dwe dasa inhale - lift the chest, (upward facing dog).

7. Trio dasa exhale - raise the hips, (downward facing dog).

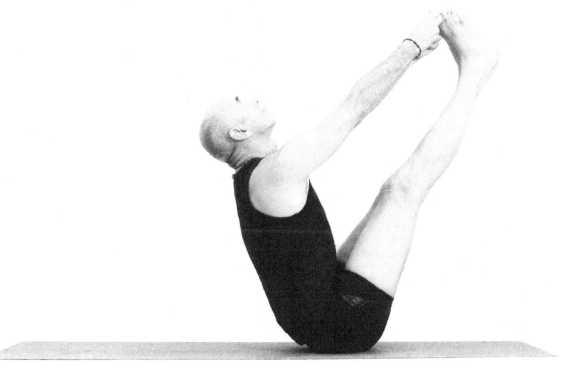

Ubhaya Padangusthasana

MODIFICATION

If you can't catch the toes, catch the ankles.

Bend the knees while coming back up.

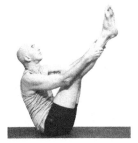

URDHVA MUKHA PACHIMATANASANA – UPWARD FACING INTENSE STRETCH

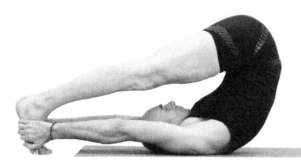

Urdhva Mukha Pachimatanasana

1. Sapta inhale - jump through to sitting, lie down exhale.

2. Hastu Inhale - take the legs back over the head, catch the heels and exhale there.

3. Nava Inhale - roll up into position, straight legs, point the toes

4. Dasa exhale - chin to knees. Take 5 breaths with sound. Dhristi big toe

5. Eka dasa inhale - straighten the arms, look up, exhale there.

6. Dwe dasa inhale – lift up

7. Trio dasa chatwari exhale - jump back to chaturanga, plank position.

8. Chatur dasa inhale - lift the chest, (upward facing dog).

9. Pancha dasa exhale - raise the hips, (downward facing dog).

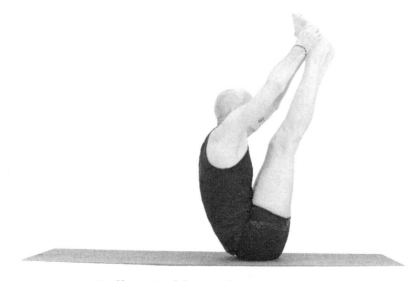

Urdhva Mukha Pachimatanasana

MODIFICATION

Bend the knees while coming back up.

If you can't catch the feet catch the ankles. See previous asana modification.

SETU BANDHASANA – SPINAL LIFT TO BRIDGE POSE

1. Sapta inhale - jump through to sitting, lie down.

2. Hastu exhale - bring the heels together open the feet, keep the legs as long as possible, bend the neck bringing the top of the head on the floor, arms crossed on the chest.

3. Nava inhale - lift hips off the ground, strong legs balancing on the head. Take 5 breaths with sound. Dhristi nose.

4. Dasa exhale - down

5. Eka dasa inhale - chakrasana, backward roll into chaturanga plank position, exhale.

6. Dwe dasa inhale - lift the chest, (upward facing dog).

7. Trio dasa exhale - raise the hips, (downward facing dog).

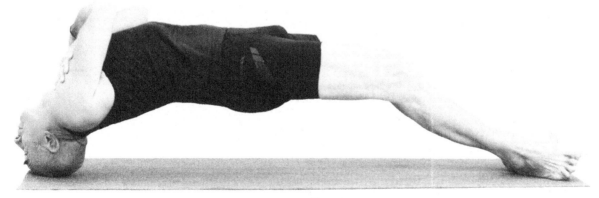

Setu Bandhasana

MODIFICATION

Support your weight with elbows on the ground when lifting up, then cross the arms on chest.

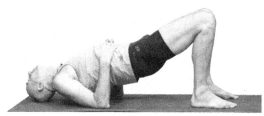

Instead of putting the weight on the head, rest on the shoulders and lift up the hip, hands can be flat or under this hips for support. Heels together open the feet.

URDHVA DANURASANA – LIFTED BOW POSE

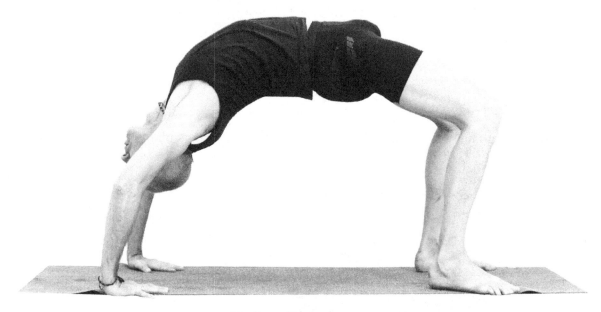

Urdhva Danurasana

1. Sapta inhale - jump through to sitting, lie down.

2. Hastu exhale - bring the feet up towards the buttocks, same width as the shoulders, bring the arms over the head elbows bent, hands facing forward.

3. Nava inhale - raise the hips and the head, while pushing down with the hands and the feet, lifting from the pelvis, do not lift the heels. Take 5 breaths with sound. Dhristi nose

4. Dasa exhale - down onto the top of the head, walk the hands in towards shoulders. Inhale lift up, Repeat total 3 times.

5. Eka dasa inhale - chakrasana backward roll into chaturanga plank position, exhale.

6. Dwe dasa inhale - lift the chest, (upward facing dog).

7. Trio dasa exhale - raise the hips, downward facing dog).

MODIFICATIONS

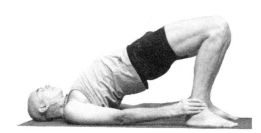

If you can't lift up the torso on the first inhale, lift up onto the top of the head, exhale there, on next inhale lift all the way up.

If you can't lift all the way up into the final position, raise the knees, bring the ankles to the hands and lift up the hips, take 5 breaths exhale down, repeat 2 more times.

PACHIMATANASANA

1. Sapta inhale- jump through to sitting straight legs, exhale.

2. Hastu inhale - catch the hands around the feet, head up.

3. Nava exhale - fold forward, lengthen the spine, Take 10 breaths with sound. Dhristi toes.

4. Dasa inhale - head up only, exhale there.

5. Eka dasa - inhale up.

6. Dwe dasa chatwari exhale - jump back to chaturanga, plank position.

7. Trio dasa inhale - lift the chest, upward facing dog.

8. Chatur dasa exhale - raise the hips, downward facing dog.

SALAMBA SARVANGASANA - SHOULDERSTANDING POSE

1. Sapta inhale- jump through to sitting, lie down, exhale.

2. Hastu inhale - raise the legs, lifting up onto the shoulders, hands placed on the lower back supporting the hips, feet together, strong legs, lifting the hips. Feet, hips, shoulders in a straight line. Take 10 breaths with sound. Dhristi nose.

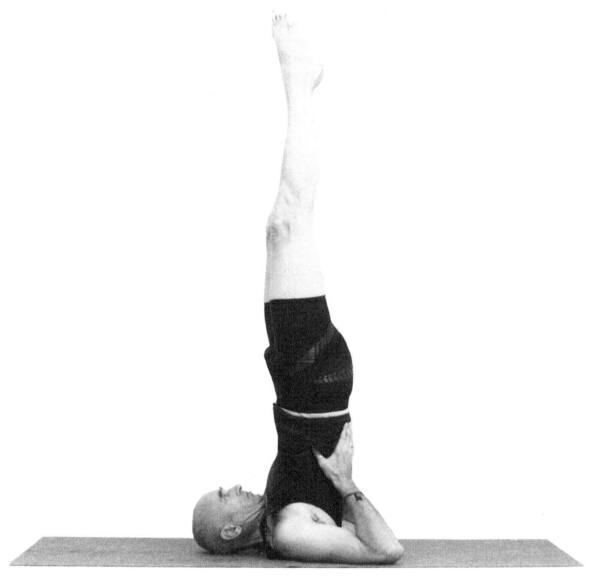

Salamba Sarvangasana

HALASANA – PLOUGH POSE

1. Hastu exhale - lower straight legs to the floor behind the head, toes pointing back, top of the toes flat on the floor, Catch hands behind the back lengthen the arms. Take 8 breaths with sound. Dhristi nose.

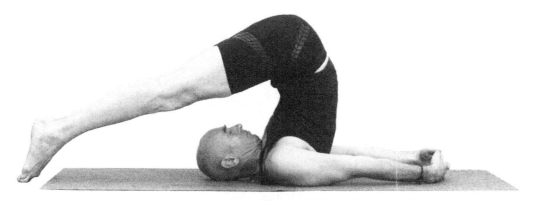

Halasana

MODIFICATION

Bend the legs slightly, support the hips if necessary.

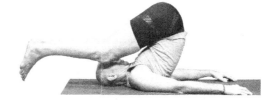

KARNA PIDASANA – EAR PRESSURE POSE

1. Hastu exhale - bend the knees closing the ears with the knees, toes pointing back, top of the toes flat on the floor, hands remain behind the back, long arms. Take 8 breaths with sound. Dhristi nose.

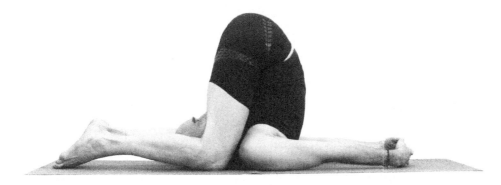

Karna Pidasana

MODIFICATION

Do not bring the knees down too far, lower to comfortable position while supporting the hips with the hands, take 5 breaths.

URDHVA PADMASANA – UPWARD LOTUS POSE

1. Nava Inhale - raise the legs, take padmasana, drop the knees to 90 degrees, hands under the knees with straight arms. Take 8 breaths with sound. Dhristi nose.

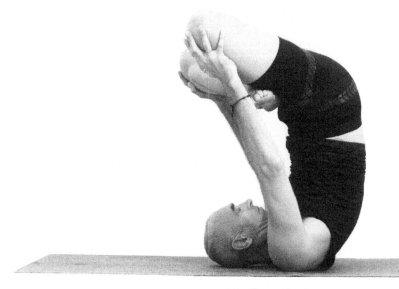

Urdhva Padmasana

MODIFICATION

If you can't do full lotus take half lotus position.

PINDASANA – EMBRYO POSE

Nava inhale - drop the knees, catch the hands together around the legs. Take 8 breaths with sound. Dhristi nose

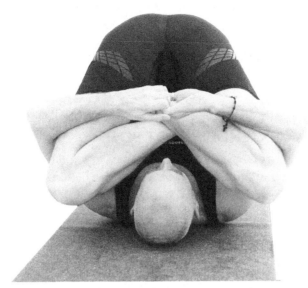

Pindasana

MODIFICATION

Lotus or half lotus, if you can't catch the hands, stretch as far around the legs as possible.

MATSYASANA – FISH POSE

Nava exhale - release the hands, roll your knees to the floor without releasing padmasana, arch the back, lift the chest, top of the head to the floor. Take 8 breaths with sound. Dhristi nose.

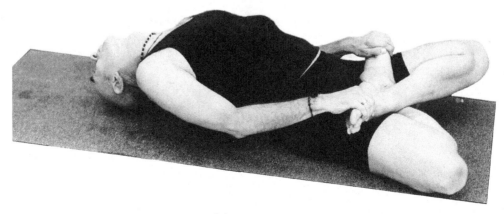

Matsyasana

MODIFICATION

If you are not in full lotus, half lotus or legs straight is acceptable.

UTTANA PADASANA – EXTENDED FOOT POSE

1. Nava exhale,- release padmasana, don't change the head position, lift straight legs to 45 degrees, raise the arms to 45 degrees, hands together. Take 8 breaths with sound. Dhristi nose.

2. Dasa inhale chakrasana - backward roll into chaturanga plank position, exhale.

3. Eka dasa inhale - lift the chest, (upward facing dog).

4. Dwe dasa exhale - raise the hips, (downward facing dog).

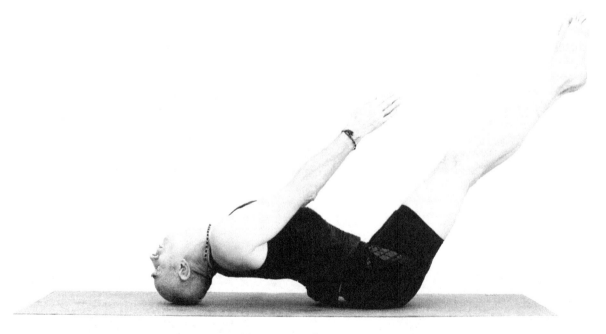

Uttana Padasana

MODIFICATION

If you are can't lift legs and arms at the same time, try lifting them individually to build strength

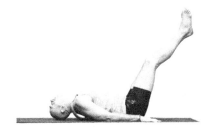 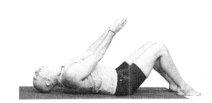

SIRSASANA – HEAD STANDING POSE (DO NOT PRACTICE SIRASANA IF YOU HAVE BP OR HEART CONDITION)

1. Sapta inhale - take position, exhale there - make a triangle with the arms, elbows forearm width apart, clasp the fingers together wrists apart making a cup to place the head down between the hands, head onto the floor. The head rests on the floor 2 to 3 inches above the hairline, (to find the right position for the head put the wrist crease on the tip of the nose, where the middle finger touches the top of the head this is the correct position)

2. Hastu inhale - walk the feet forward hips above the shoulders, lift into position. Straight legs, feet together point the toes. Ankles, hips, shoulders, wrists should be in a straight line. Take 15 breaths with sound. Dhristi nose.

3. Nava exhale - drop the legs to 90 degrees strong legs, feet pointing forward. Take 10 breaths with sound. Dhristi nose.

4. Inhale, lift the legs back up to sirasana position. Take 10 breaths with sound. Dhristi nose.

5. Dasa exhale - legs down to the floor slowly, take child pose without changing the head position. Take 10 breaths with sound.

6. Eka dasa chatwari exhale - jump back to chaturanga, plank position.

7. Dwe dasa inhale - lift the chest, (upward facing dog).

8. Trio dasa exhale - raise the hips, (downward facing dog).

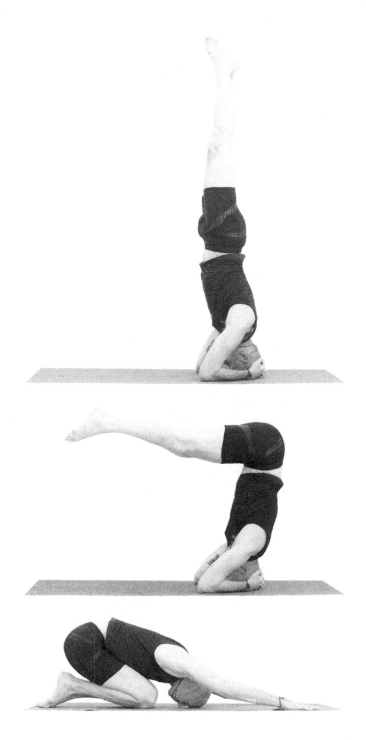

Sirsasana

YOGA AND DIET CURED MY ARTHRITIS · 141

MODIFICATION

Hastu inhale, walk the feet and hips forward, bring one knee to chest, lift, next bring both knees to chest, and breathe there. First get used to this position before trying to extend fully, this is still a headstand but with no fear. When you are ready extend the legs.

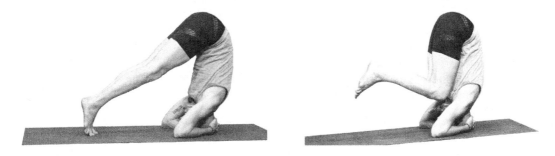

BADDHA PADMASANA – BOUND LOTUS POSE

1. Sapta inhale - jump through to sitting, exhale.

2. Hastu inhale -take padmasana, bring the left hand round the back and catch the left big toe, take right hand round the back and catch the right big toe.

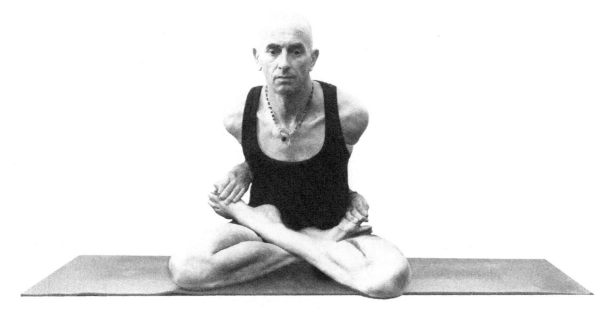

Baddha Padmasana

MODIFICATION

Catch the elbows instead of the feet, or use towels to
catch the feet, exhale down.

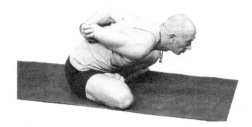

YOGA MUDRA A – SACRED SEAL

3. Nava exhale - bend forward, lengthen the spine, chin to the floor. Take 10 breaths
with sound. Dhristi nose

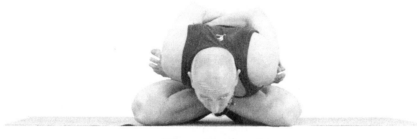

Yoga Mudra A

YOGA MUDRA B

4. Dasa Inhale - come back up, take the hands back about 12 inches behind the hips,
raise the chest, head back. Take 10 breaths with sound. Dhristi nose.

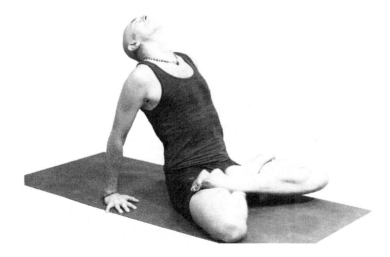

Yoga Mudra B

PADMASANA – FULL LOTUS POSE

5. Dasa inhale - raise the head, take hand mudra. Straight back, drop the chin, all 3 bandhas engaged. Take 10 breaths with sound. Dhristi nose.

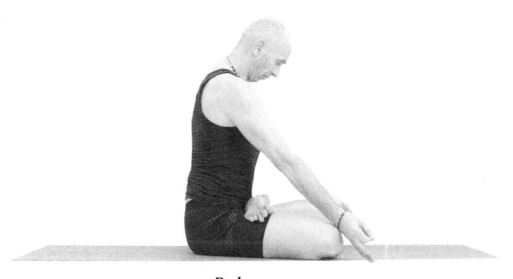

Padmasana

UTPLUTIH – SCALES POSE

6. Dasa inhale up - hands on the floor at the side of the waist, lift the knees, draw the body upwards from mula bandha. Take 10 breaths with sound. Dhristi nose.

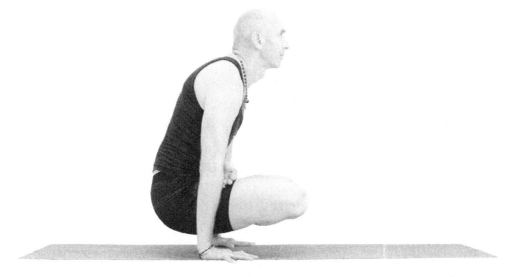

Utplutih

MODIFICATION

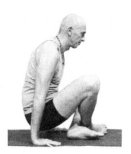

If you are not in full lotus, half lotus is acceptable, lift up, keeping the buttocks off the floor.

8. Eka dasa chatwari exhale - jump back to chaturanga plank position.

9. Dwe dasa inhale - lift the chest, (upward facing dog).

10. Trio dasa - exhale raise the hips, (downward facing dog).

11. Chatur dasa inhale - jump forward head up.

12. Pancha dasa exhale - drop the head.

13. Sho dasa inhale - come to standing, stretch tall hands above the head. Exhale release. Samasthiti

Bring the hands together in prayer position.

CLOSING MANTRA

Om
Svasti prajabhya pari pala yantam nyayena margena mahim mahisah,
Gobramanebhyah subha mastu nityam lokah samastah sukhino bhavantu
Om santih, santih, santih

Translation

May all be well with mankind,
May the leaders of the earth protect in every way by keeping to the right path.
May there be goodness for those who know the earth to be sacred,
May all the worlds be happy.

1. Ekam inhale – raise the arms stretch tall lifting from the elbows extending the armpits and sides.

2. Dwe exhale – fold forward from the hips, extending the hands to the floor.

3. Trini inhale – head up only.

4. Chatwari exhale – jump back to chaturanga plank position.

5. Pancha inhale – raise the chest look up, (upward facing dog).

6. Sapta exhale – raise the hips, (downward facing dog).

7. Shat inhale – jump forward straight legs sit down, lay down take rest, shavasana position 10 minutes.

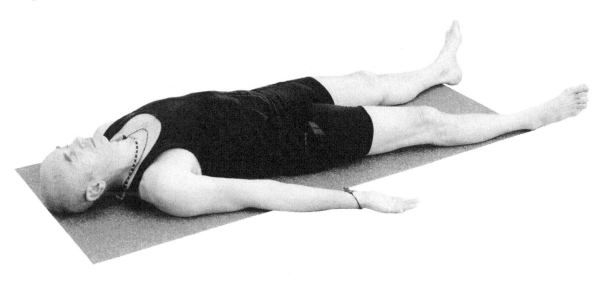

Relax, observe the breath, enjoy this time and the end of your asana practice.

SECTION 7: PRIMARY SERIES CHEAT SHEET

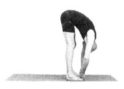

padangusthasana

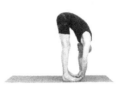

pada hastasana

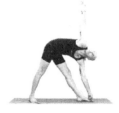

utthita trikonasana A

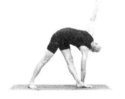

utthita trikonasana B

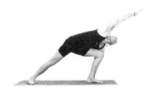

utthita parsvakonasana A

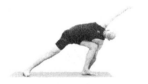

utthita parsvakonasana B

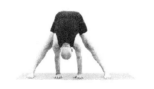

prasarita padottanasana A

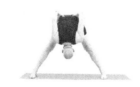

prasarita padottanasana B

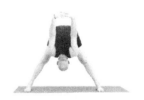

prasarita padottanasana C

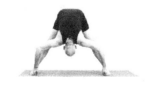

prasarita padottanasana D

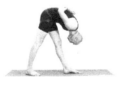

parsvottanasana

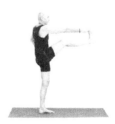

utthita hasta padangusthasana A

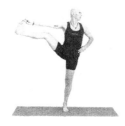

utthita hasta padangusthasana B

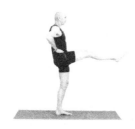

utthita hasta padangusthasana C

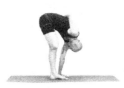

ardha badha padmottanasana

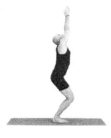

utkatasana

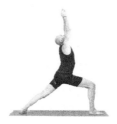

virabhadrasana A

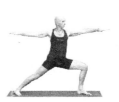

virabhadrasana B

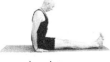

dandasana

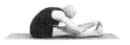

paschimattanasana A

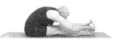

paschimattanasana B

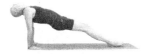

purvattanasana

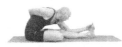

ardha badha padma
paschimattanasana

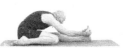

triang mukha ekapada
paschimattanasana

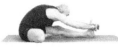

janusirsasana A

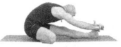

janusirsasana B

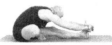

janusirsasana C

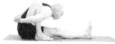

marichasana A

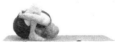

marichasana B

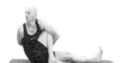

marichasana C

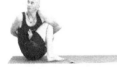

maricasana D

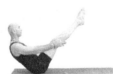

navasana

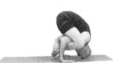

bhujapidasana

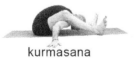

kurmasana

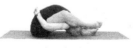

supta kurmasana

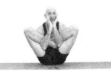

garbha pindasana

kukkutasana

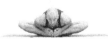

baddha konasana A

baddha konasana B

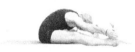

upavistha konasana A

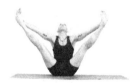

upavistha konasana B

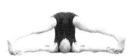

supta konasana

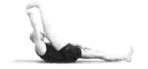

supta padangusthasana A

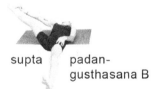

supta padan-
gusthasana B

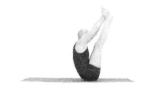

ubhaya padangusthasana

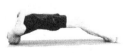

urdhvamukha pascimattanasana

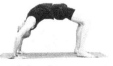

setu bandhasana

urdvha danurasana

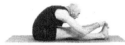

pascimattanasana

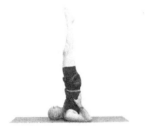

salamba sarvangasana

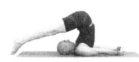

halasana

karna pidasana

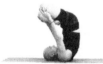

urdhva padmasana

pindasana

matsyasana

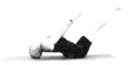

uttana padasana

sirsasana

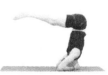

sirsasana B

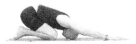

balasana (child pose)

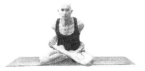

baddha padmasana

yoga mudra A

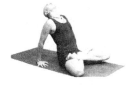

yoga mudra B

padmasana

utpluthi

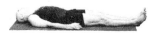

savasana - take rest

SECTION 8: VINYASA, CHAKRASANA, PADMASANA

I refer to vinyasa in this context as both the transition into and the exit from asana.

JUMPING THROUGH

From downward facing dog position:

1. Inhale - bandhas engaged, gazing point should be in front of your hands, ahead of where you intend to land your feet. Bend the knees and jump the hips with a upward trajectory with straight legs (try not to kick out your legs like a donkey). If you lead with the hips, the legs will follow. When you reach the top of the jump, tuck the sitting bones under, lowering and crossing the legs, bringing them through the hands to sitting position.

Some people come through with straight legs, some people with crossed legs, both are correct, the key is strong bandha.

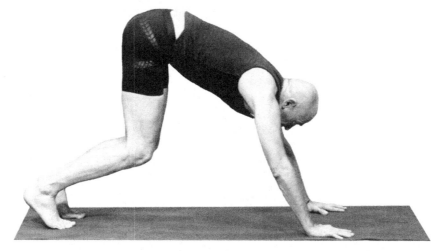

Jumping Through

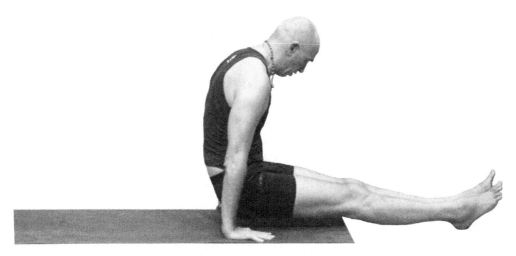

Jumping Through

MODIFICATIONS

If you can't jump the legs through, don't worry; your arms are not too short! In time with dedicated practice and bandha, it will come. Try this:

1. Inhale - jump the feet between the hands as far as possible, now continue to walk through the hands without raising the wrists off the floor, straighten the legs then lower down.

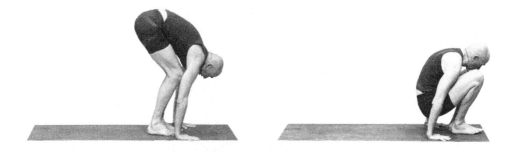

Remember to look ahead of where you expect your feet to land.

If the jump through is too difficult you can walk forward from downward facing dog, trying to bring the feet through the hands before sitting.

ONE YEAR CHALLENGE:

Get 2 books each with around 300 to 400 pages, place your hands on the books and jump through as if you were using blocks. Each day rip out one page from each book and within a year you will be jumping through without assistance.

You can also use the books to learn the 'lift up', drawing the energy up with bandha as in vinyasa and Utplutih.

JUMPING BACK

As you finish the asanas from sitting position.

1. Inhale – lift up, bring the hands to the floor, legs crossed to allow jump back.

2. Chatwari exhale - jump or walk back to chaturanga, plank position.

3. Inhale - raise the chest (upward facing dog).

4. Exhale - raise the hips (downward facing dog).

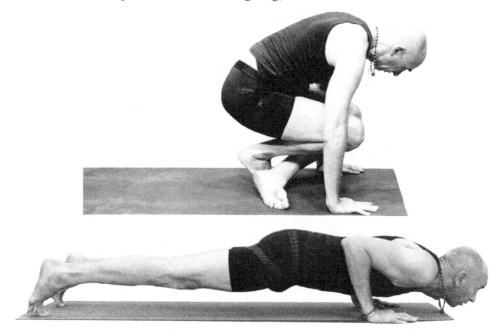

Jumping Back
Advanced practitioners will usually exit vinyasa the following way.

1. Inhale – lift up, balancing on the hands, legs crossed above the ankle, knees to chest.

2. Chatwari exhale - lower the head towards the floor without touching the floor with your feet, Swing your legs back and through the arms, straight legs to Chaturanga Dandasana (plank position).

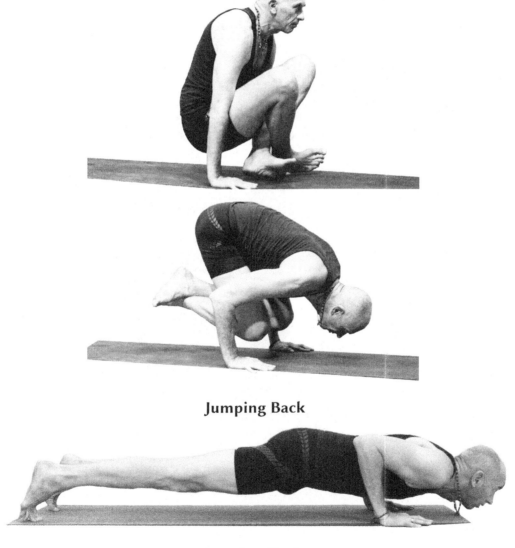

Jumping Back

Jumping Back

Again the secret to this vinyasa movement and transfer of weight is bandha. Keep checking your bandha. Strong bandha; light body. 'practice, practice all is coming' (K.P.Jois.)

CHAKRASANA

1. Lying back down, bring the hands behind the shoulders, palms down fingers pointing toward the feet.

2. Inhale - Bring your legs back, knees to chest and over the head, press the hands down into the floor and let the momentum and the weight of the hips take you back.

3. Exhale - as you land in chaturanga, plank position.

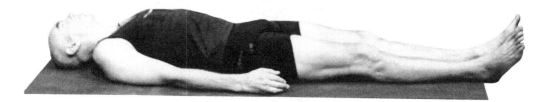

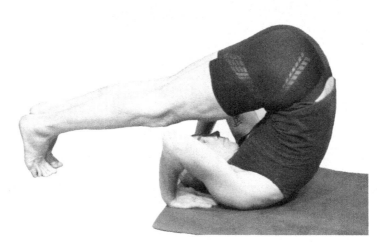

Chakrasana

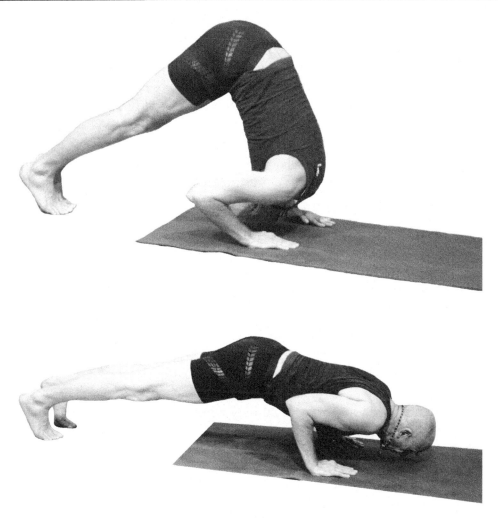

Chakrasana

MODIFICATION

Bring the hands behind the shoulders, fingers pointing toward the feet.

Inhale - Bring your legs back, knees to chest and over the head, press the hands down into the floor and roll over on one shoulder.

By practicing this way you will learn to experience the 'lift' from pressing down with the hands, eventually learning to lift and roll back over the head without fear of hurting your neck.

PADMASANA

Padmasana is often the first big challenge when most people start yoga. Through the western habit of sitting in chairs our hips are often very closed. I see many students in my workshops who could very easily sit in padmasana but they do not know the correct technique to attain it.

1. Sit with straight legs and straight back bandhas engaged. Inhale raise the right knee pulling the heel as close to your buttocks as possible safely stretching the knee.

2. Exhale let the right knee fall out to the side opening the hip.

3. Inhale bring the right heel up towards the naval, keep the foot pointing forward engaged.

4. Exhale, keeping the foot as high as possible on the thigh, allow the knee to relax down, open the calf muscle.

5. Inhale bring the left leg into position.

Hold padmasana comfortably with awareness of the breath.

If you feel too much discomfort, release and try again, slowly increase the length of time you can sit each day without strain, over time it will feel natural to sit this way.

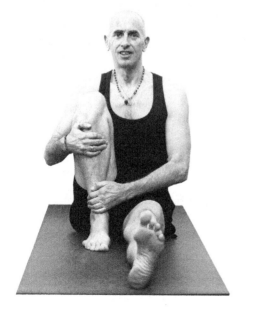 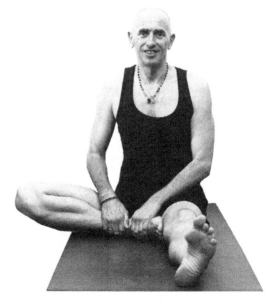

Padmasana

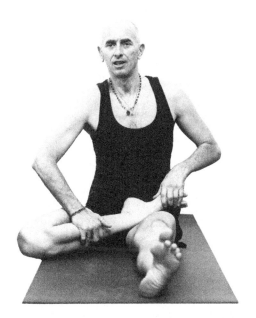 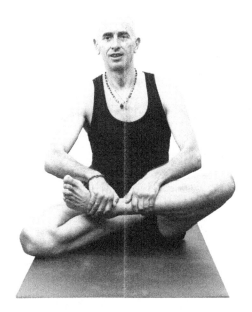

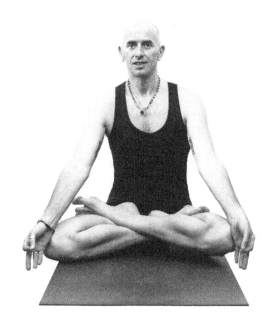

Padmasana

APPENDIX 1: LEARNING YOGA - MYSORE STYLE

WHAT IS MYSORE STYLE?

'Mysore Style' is the traditional way to learn Ashtanga Yoga as taught by Sri K. Pattabhi Jois RIP and since then by his daughter Saraswathi and his grandson R. Sharath Jois in Mysore, India.

The series of asana is learnt at each individual's own speed and capacity, starting off with Suryanamaskar A & B, the Sun Salutations which builds the foundation. Then more asanas are added step-by-step, which enables you to learn each posture individually and in the correct method. In the beginning the practice takes less time but gradually it becomes more intense, building to the full series. With the correct guidance your teacher will lead you through the series and you will develop a practice of meditation in motion.

Progress comes from regular practice only. As Sri K. Pattabhi Jois famously said:

"Practice, practice, all is coming" and "99% practice; 1% theory"

BENEFITS OF THIS METHOD OF LEARNING YOGA

Yoga Asana is a practice for yourself, for your own development. "Mysore Style" allows this. You start to practice and slowly your own personal practice develops. Everybody is different; this is why the Yoga practice should also be different and individual.

WHAT DOES A MYSORE CLASS LOOK LIKE?

Beginners and advanced practitioners practice next to each other, each one in their own rhythm. By observing other practitioners you can learn the sequence. Everybody follows the same set sequence. Silence is another noticeable factor, other than the constant noise of the unifying ujayi breath of the practitioners.

How to behave in a Mysore Class:

• Remove your footwear. Only bring things into the practice room that you need for your practice. No water bottles.

• Hygiene is essential, if you practice Yoga your clothes as well as your mat and body should be clean.

• Don't eat anything for 2 hours before your practice.

• Class starts with chanting the opening mantra. If you arrive late, start the opening mantra in silence.

• Follow the given sequence of the asana. Don't bring the asana cheat sheet.

• Always inform the teacher about any injuries or physical difficulties.

• Don't enter a new asana until your teacher gives it to you. Don't ask for a new asana, everything will come at the right time.

• If you need an adjustment, and the teacher is helping another student, wait patiently until the teacher is free.

• Stay on your own mat and don't adjust other students.

• Practice within your limitations, wait for the openings to happen, enjoy the journey of the breath.

• Don't talk. Keep silence in the practice room.

MYSORE LED PRACTICE

Twice weekly in Mysore Sharath Jois leads a Mysore led practice, where all the students start at the same time and move in unison through the whole series following Sharath's vinyasa count in Sanskrit as detailed earlier.

The full practice with opening and closing mantra is approximately 1 hour and 20 minutes.

When Sharath is on his international tours he usually leads a led class each morning for 6 continuous days.

APPENDIX 2: GLOSSARY OF TERMS

This glossary contains terms and concepts used in this document. Only some key Hindu and Sanskrit words and concepts are translated or explained.

Unless otherwise stated definitions and explanations are sourced from the Oxford online dictionary

https://en.oxforddictionaries.com

or from the MedicineNet medical dictionary website

http://www.medicinenet.com/medterms-medical-dictionary/article.htm.

Term or concept	Definition or explanation
Acupuncture	A system of complementary medicine in which fine needles are inserted in the skin at specific points along lines of energy (meridians).
Alexander technique	A system designed to promote well-being by retraining one's awareness and habits of posture to ensure minimum effort and strain.
Alkaline foods	The science of alkaline foods recognizes that elements and compounds in food cause different reactions in our body when digested. Some elements, for example, proteins and phosphorous produce acidic salts. Other elements, e.g. potassium, magnesium and calcium, produce alkaline salts. These salts end up at our kidneys, where they alter the pH environment. This process has resulted in the Potential

	Renal Acid Load (PRAL) calculation, which is an approximate estimate of the effect of foods on the acidity/alkalinity of our bodies. Or more specifically, of urine, as this is the measurable result. http://www.goutpal.com/810/alkaline-foods-more-myths-exposed/
Alternative therapy	Alternative medicine practices are used instead of standard medical treatments. Alternative medicine is distinct from complementary medicine, which is meant to accompany, not to replace, standard medical practices.
Antibiotics	A medicine (such as penicillin or its derivatives) that inhibits the growth of or destroys microorganisms.
Anti-inflammatory	A drug used to reduce inflammation.
Arthritis	A disease causing painful inflammation and stiffness of the joints.
Asana	From Sanskrit āsana seat, manner of sitting. A posture adopted in performing hatha yoga.
Ashtanga yoga (astanga)	A type of yoga based on eight principles and consisting of a series of poses executed in swift succession, vinyasa, combined with deep, controlled breathing, bandha body locks and Dristhi gazing point. From Hindi aṣṭan or its source, Sanskrit ashṭaṅga having eight parts, from ashtán eight.
Aum, Ohm, Om.	A mystic syllable, considered the most sacred mantra in Hinduism and Tibetan Buddhism. It appears at the beginning and end of most Sanskrit recitations, prayers, and texts.
Ayurveda/Ayurvedic	The traditional Hindu system of medicine, which is based on the idea of balance in bodily systems and uses diet, herbal treatment, and yogic breathing.
Bandha	Body lock (in yoga).

Braise	Fry food lightly and then stew it slowly in a closed container.
Carbohydrate	Any of a large group of organic compounds occurring in foods and living tissues and including sugars, starch, and cellulose. They can be broken down to release energy in the body.
Cartilage	Firm, flexible connective tissue found in various forms in the larynx and respiratory tract, in structures such as the external ear, and in the articulating surfaces of joints.
Circulation	The continuous motion by which the blood travels through all parts of the body under the action of the heart.
Cod liver oil	Oil pressed from the liver of cod, rich in vitamins D and A.
Crustacean	An arthropod of the large aquatic group, such as a crab, lobster, or shrimp.
Cure	Relieve a person of the symptoms of a disease or condition.
Diet	A special course of food to which a person restricts themselves, either to lose weight or for medical reasons.
Dristhi	Gazing point (in yoga).
Drug	A medicine or other substance that has a physiological effect when ingested or otherwise introduced into the body.
E numbers	E numbers are codes for substances that are permitted for use as food additives within the European Union and other jurisdictions. For more information and the list of E numbers: https://en.wikipedia.org/wiki/E_number
Essential oil	An oil derived from a natural substance, usually either for its healing properties or as a perfume.
Evidence-based medicine	The judicious use of the best current available scientific research in making decisions about the care of patients. Evidence-based medicine (EBM) is intended to integrate clinical expertise with the research evidence and patient values.

Food combinations	Food combining (also known as trophology) is a term for a nutritional approach that advocates specific combinations of foods as central to good health and weight loss (such as not mixing carbohydrate-rich foods and protein-rich foods in the same meal).
Glaucoma	A common eye condition in which the fluid pressure inside the eye rises to a level higher than healthy for that eye.
Glucosamine, Chondroitin	A molecule derived from the sugar glucose by the addition of an amino group. Glucosamine is a component of a number of structures, including the blood group substances and cartilage. Glucosamine is currently in use as a nutritional supplement (often in combination with chondroitin) and is touted as a remedy for arthritic symptoms.
Gout	A disease in which defective metabolism of uric acid causes arthritis, especially in the smaller bones of the feet, deposition of chalk-stones, and episodes of acute pain.
Growth hormone	A hormone which stimulates growth in animal or plant cells, especially (in animals) that is secreted by the pituitary gland.
Guru	A Hindu spiritual teacher.
Hatha yoga	The branch of yoga which concentrates on physical health and mental well-being through postures (asanas), breathing techniques (pranayama), and meditation (dyana) http://medical-dictionary.thefreedictionary.com/hatha+yoga
Hatha Yoga Pradipika	The Hatha Yoga Pradīpikā) is a classic Sanskrit manual on hatha yoga, written by Svāmi Svātmārāma, a disciple of Swami Gorakhnath in the 15th Century. https://en.wikipedia.org/wiki/Hatha_Yoga_Pradipika
Homeopathy	A system of complementary medicine in which ailments are treated by minute doses of natural substances that in larger amounts would produce symptoms of the ailment.

Hormones	A chemical substance produced in the body that controls and regulates the activity of certain cells or organs. Hormones are essential for every activity of life, including the processes of digestion, metabolism, growth, reproduction, and mood control. Many hormones, such as neurotransmitters, are active in more than one physical process.
Ibuprofen	A synthetic compound used widely as an analgesic and anti-inflammatory drug.
Immune system	A complex system that is responsible for distinguishing a person from everything foreign to him or her and for protecting the body against infections and foreign substances.
Inflammation	A localized physical condition in which part of the body becomes reddened, swollen, hot, and often painful, especially as a reaction to injury or infection.
Infusion	A drink, remedy, or extract prepared by soaking leaves or herbs in liquid.
Iyengar yoga / BKS Iyengar	A type of Hatha yoga focusing on the correct alignment of the body, making use of straps, wooden blocks, and other objects as aids in achieving the correct postures. BKS Iyengar was also a student of Krishnamacharya.
Jumping back and through	See Vinyassa
Karma	In Hinduism and Buddhism the sum of a person's actions in this and previous states of existence, viewed as deciding their fate in future existences.
KPJAYI	Krishna Pattabhi Jois Ashtanga Yoga Institute (Mysore India)
Mainstream medicine	Medicine as practiced by holders of degrees in medicine or surgery and by their allied health professionals, such as physical therapists, psychologists, and registered nurses. The term "mainstream medicine" implies that other forms of treatment, such as 'alternative therapies', are outside the mainstream.

Medicine/medication	A drug or other preparation for the treatment or prevention of disease.
Meditate	To focus one's mind for a period of time, in silence or with the aid of chanting, for religious or spiritual purposes or as a method of relaxation.
Mineral	An inorganic substance needed by the human body for good health.
Mindfulness	A mental state achieved by focusing one's awareness on the present moment, while calmly acknowledging and accepting one's feelings, thoughts, and bodily sensations, used as a therapeutic technique.
Mudra	A symbolic or ritual hand gesture.
National health system (NHS)	The United Kingdom's publicly funded health system.
Naturopathy	A system of alternative medicine based on the theory that diseases can be successfully treated or prevented without the use of drugs, by techniques such as control of diet, exercise, and massage.
Nausea	A feeling of sickness with an inclination to vomit.
Nutrient, nutritious, nourishing	A substance that provides nourishment essential for the maintenance of life and for growth.
Omega 3 fatty acid	An unsaturated fatty acid occurring chiefly in fish oils.
Organic	Of food or farming methods produced or involving production without the use of chemical fertilizers, pesticides, or other artificial chemicals.
Osteoarthritis	Degeneration of joint cartilage and the underlying bone, most common from middle age onward. It causes pain and stiffness, especially in the hip, knee, and thumb joints.

Pain gateways	The gate control theory of pain asserts that non-painful input closes the "gates" to painful input, which prevents pain sensation from traveling to the central nervous system. Therefore, stimulation by non-noxious input is able to suppress pain. https://en.wikipedia.org/wiki/Gate_control_theory
Pranayama	In yoga, the conscious and careful regulation of breath.
Prescribe	Advise and authorize the use of (a medicine or treatment) for someone, especially in writing.
Processed foods	The term 'processed food' applies to any food that has been altered from its natural state in some way, either for safety reasons or convenience. Food processing techniques include freezing, canning, baking, drying and pasteurising products. http://www.nhs.uk/Livewell/Goodfood/Pages/what-are-processed-foods.aspx For more info see: http://www.eatright.org/resource/food/nutrition/nutrition-facts-and-food-labels/avoiding-processed-foods
Protein	Nitrogenous organic compounds which are an essential part of all living organisms, especially as structural components of body tissues such as muscle, hair, etc., and as enzymes and antibodies.
Refined grains	Refining grains removes varying proportions of the bran and germ. Because micronutrients are generally present in higher concentrations in these outer layers of the grain, refined grain products are lower in vitamins and minerals than whole grains. For more information see: http://www.glnc.org.au/grains/grains-and-nutrition/refined-grains/
Repetitive stress syndrome or injury	An injury that occurs due to recurrent overuse or improper use of a limb or joint.

Restrict	Put a limit on; keep under control.
Rheumatoid arthritis	A chronic progressive disease causing inflammation in the joints and resulting in painful deformity and immobility, especially in the fingers, wrists, feet, and ankles.
Smoothie	A thick, smooth drink of fresh fruit pureed with milk, yogurt, or ice cream.
Solanaceae, nightshade	Solanaceae, or nightshades, are a family of flowering plants. Many members of the family contain potent alkaloids, and some are highly toxic, but many cultures eat nightshades, in some cases as staple foods. https://en.wikipedia.org/wiki/Solanaceae
Steroid	A class of organic compounds with a characteristic molecular structure including many hormones, alkaloids, and vitamins.
Stress	A state of mental or emotional strain or tension resulting from adverse or demanding circumstances.
Supine	Lying face upwards.
Supplement	A thing added to something else in order to complete or enhance it.
Suppress	Prevent the development, action, or expression of (a feeling, impulse, idea, disease etc.); restrain.
Suryanamaskar or Surya Namaskar	Sun salutation
Symptom	A physical or mental feature indicating a condition of disease.
Synovial membrane	A layer of connective tissue that lines the cavities of joints, tendon sheaths, and bursae and makes synovial fluid, which has a lubricating function.
Therapeutic modality	An intervention used to heal someone.
Tonic	A medicinal substance taken to give a feeling of vigour or well-being.

Trans fats	Trans fats are uncommon in nature but may be found in low levels in beef, lamb and dairy foods. Processed foods can contain larger amounts of trans fats due to manufacturing processes or from superheating oils and fats during food production. Foods that may contain higher levels of trans fats include: Deep fried foods, commercial cakes and biscuits, pies and pastries. http://daa.asn.au/for-the-public/smart-eating-for-you/nutrition-a-z/trans-fats/
Ujayi breath	Breathing with sound (in ashtanga yoga).
Uric acid	A breakdown product of purines that are part of many foods. In gout, there are frequently, but not always, elevated levels of uric acid in the blood (hyperuricemia).
Vinyassa	A vinyasa, in essence, consists of moving from one asana, or body position, to another, combining breathing with the movement. The Surya Namaskar and each of the successive asanas are comprised of a particular number of vinyasas. http://kpjayi.org/the-practice/traditional-method/
Vipasana	In Theravada Buddhism - meditation involving concentration on the body or its sensations, or the insight which this provides.
Vitamin	Any of a group of organic compounds that are essential for normal growth and nutrition and are required in small quantities in the diet because they cannot be synthesized by the body.
Whole grain	Describes an intact grain, flour or a food that contains all three parts of the grain. For more information see: http://www.glnc.org.au/grains/grains-and-nutrition/wholegrains/

Ying Yang	Yin (in Chinese philosophy) the passive female principle of the universe, characterized as sustaining and associated with earth, dark and cold. Yang (in Chinese philosophy) the active male principle of the universe, characterized as creative and associated with heaven, heat and light.
Yoga	Yoga is a group of physical, mental, and spiritual practices or disciplines that originated in ancient India. There is a broad variety of Yoga schools, practices, and goals. In Vedic Sanskrit, yoga (from the root yuj) means "to add", "to join", "to unite", or "to attach" in its most common literal sense.
Yogi, yogin, yogini	Someone who practices yoga or follows the yoga philosophy with a high level of commitment. https://en.wikipedia.org/wiki/Yoga
Zen	A Japanese school of Mahayana Buddhism emphasizing the value of meditation and intuition rather than ritual worship or study of scriptures.

SANSKRIT NUMBERS

1 – Ekam

2 – Dwe

3 – Trini

4 – Chatwari

5 – Pancha

6 – Shat

7 – Sapta

8 – Hastu

9 – Nava

10 – Dasa

11 – Eka dasa

12 – Dwe dasa

13 – Trio dasa

14 – Chatur dasa

15 – Pancha dasa

16 – Sho dasa

17 – Sapta dasa

18 – Hastu dasa

19 – Ekona Vimshatih

20 – Vimshatih

21 – Eka vimshatih

22 – Dwe vimshatih

23 – Trio vimshatih

24 – Chatur vimshatih

25 – Pancha vimshatih

26 – Shat vimshatih

27 – Sapta vimshatih

28 – Hastu vimshatih

29 – Ekona Trimshat

30 – Trimshat

AUTHOR BIO

Mark Flint was diagnosed with rheumatoid arthritis over 25 years ago. He had always been fit and athletic, an ex-professional golfer and successful businessman. When diagnosed he was advised to take a steroid a day for the rest of his life or end up in a wheel-chair. He chose not to take this advice. Instead, he went on a course of discovery about how to put his body back together without resorting to medications. He began by experimenting with foods to find an arthritis friendly diet and trying various other alternative remedies and treatments.

Born and raised in the UK Mark now lives in Mysore India with his wife Stephanie and young son Oliver. There they run a heritage guesthouse 'Shanti Nilayam' have a business making yoga accessories and also teach yoga around Asia for several months each year. It is in Mysore that Mark discovered the benefits of a regular yoga practice to his condition. He began practicing yoga in 1999 and later moved on to the ashtanga yoga system under the guidance of Sharath and Saraswathi Jois in 2009. In 2012 Mark was authorised by the K. Pattabhi Jois Ashtanga Institute to teach this style of traditional ashtanga yoga.

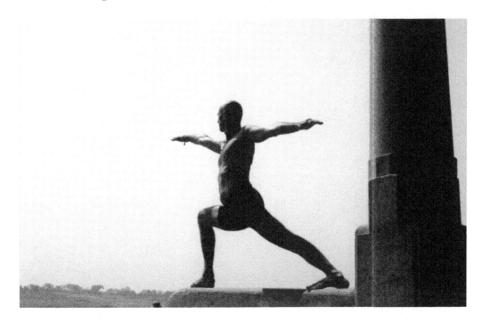

Thank you for reading my book, if you enjoyed it please take a moment and leave me a review at your favourite retailer.

http://www.yoganaddietcuredmyarthritis.com

http://www.markflintyoga.org

email: ifa_international@hotmail.com

Whatsapp 00919880148055

Instagram: Yorkshire_buddha

Wechat: markflintyoga

Thank You Mark

Made in the USA
Monee, IL
21 May 2022

96842075R10098